The Affordable Vegan Air Fryer Meals

On a Budget Recipes for your Daily Meals

Samantha Attanasio

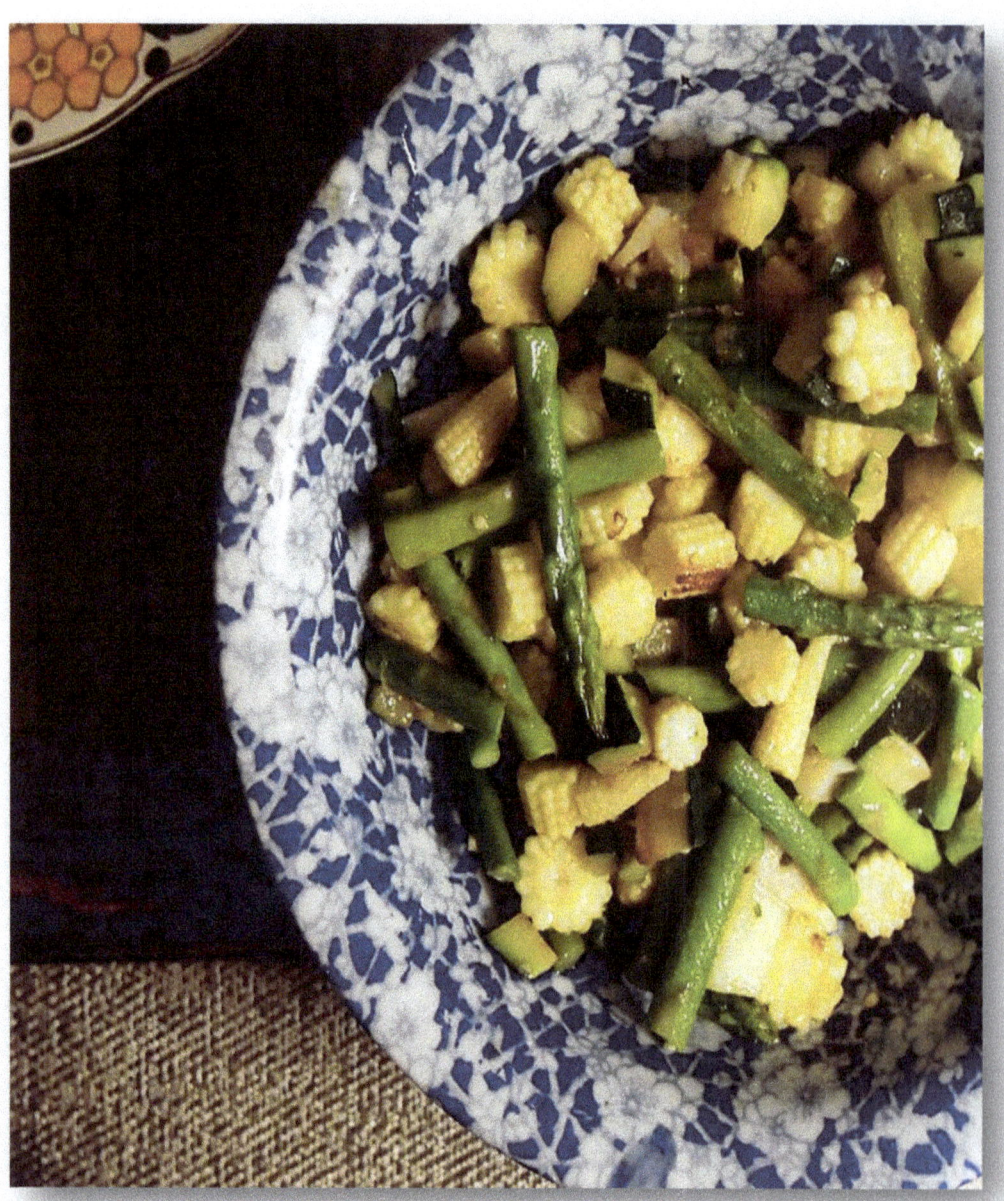

© copyright 2021 – all rights reserved.

the content contained within this book may not be reproduced, duplicated or transmitted without direct written permission from the author or the publisher.

under no circumstances will any blame or legal responsibility be held against the publisher, or author, for any damages, reparation, or monetary loss due to the information contained within this book. either directly or indirectly.

legal notice:

this book is copyright protected. this book is only for personal use. you cannot amend, distribute, sell, use, quote or paraphrase any part, or the content within this book, without the consent of the author or publisher.

disclaimer notice:

please note the information contained within this document is for educational and entertainment purposes only. all effort has been executed to present accurate, up to date, and reliable, complete information. no warranties of any kind are declared or implied. readers acknowledge that the author is not engaging in the rendering of legal, financial, medical or professional advice. the content within this book has been derived from various sources. please consult a licensed professional before attempting any techniques outlined in this book.

by reading this document, the reader agrees that under no circumstances is the author responsible for any losses, direct or indirect, which are incurred as a result of the use of information contained within this document, including, but not limited to, — errors, omissions, or inaccuracies.

Table of Contents

VEGETABLE 7

    LEMON ARTICHOKES 7

    ORANGE LAVA CAKE 9

    CINNAMON APPLES 11

    CARROT AND PINEAPPLE CINNAMON BREAD 13

    COCOA AND COCONUT BARS 15

    VANILLA CAKE 17

    SWEET APPLE CUPCAKES 19

    ORANGE BREAD WITH ALMONDS 22

    TANGERINE CAKE 24

    MAPLE TOMATO BREAD 26

    LEMON SQUARES 28

    DATES AND CASHEW STICKS 30

    GRAPE PUDDING 32

    COCONUT AND PUMPKIN SEEDS BARS 34

    CINNAMON BANANAS 36

    COFFEE PUDDING 38

    BLUEBERRY CAKE 40

    PEACH CINNAMON COBBLER 42

VEGAN FRUITS 44

    CARAMELIZED BANANAS 44

    PREPARATION TIME: 10 MINUTES 44

    BANANA ROLLS 45

    FRIED OMELET OF RIPE BANANAS 47

    SWEET CORN PIES 48

BANANA PIE	50
APPLE FRITTERS	52
FRIED APPLES	53
BANANA SALAD	54
SALAD OF RICE AND AVOCADOS	56

VEGAN DESSERT 58

TOMATO CAKE	58
BERRIES MIX	60
PASSION FRUIT PUDDING	62
PUMPKIN COOKIES	64
FIGS AND COCONUT BUTTER MIX	66
PEARS AND ESPRESSO CREAM	67
CHOCOLATE CHIP COOKIES	69
OATMEAL RAISIN COOKIES	72
EASY CINNAMON CRISPS	75
DE-LIGHT-FULL CARAMELIZED APPLES	77

VEGAN SNACKS 79

BEETS CHIPS	79
AVOCADO CHIPS	80
VEGGIE STICKS	82
POLENTA BISCUITS	84

VEGAN BREAD AND PIZZA 85

BANANA CHOCOLATE MUFFINS	85
VEGAN CORN BREAD	87
VEGAN BANANA BREAD	89
VEGAN BREAD WITH LENTILS AND UNLEAVENED MILLET	91

VEGAN MAIN DISHES 93

THE EASY PANEER PIZZA 93

CAULIFLOWER SAUCE AND PASTA 95

TAMARIND GLAZED SWEET POTATOES 97

VEGAN STAPLES 99

THAI-INSPIRED BARBECUE CAULIFLOWER 99

STUFFED GARLIC MUSHROOMS 101

STICKY MUSHROOM RICE 103

CRISPY TOFU 105

Vegetable

Lemon Artichokes

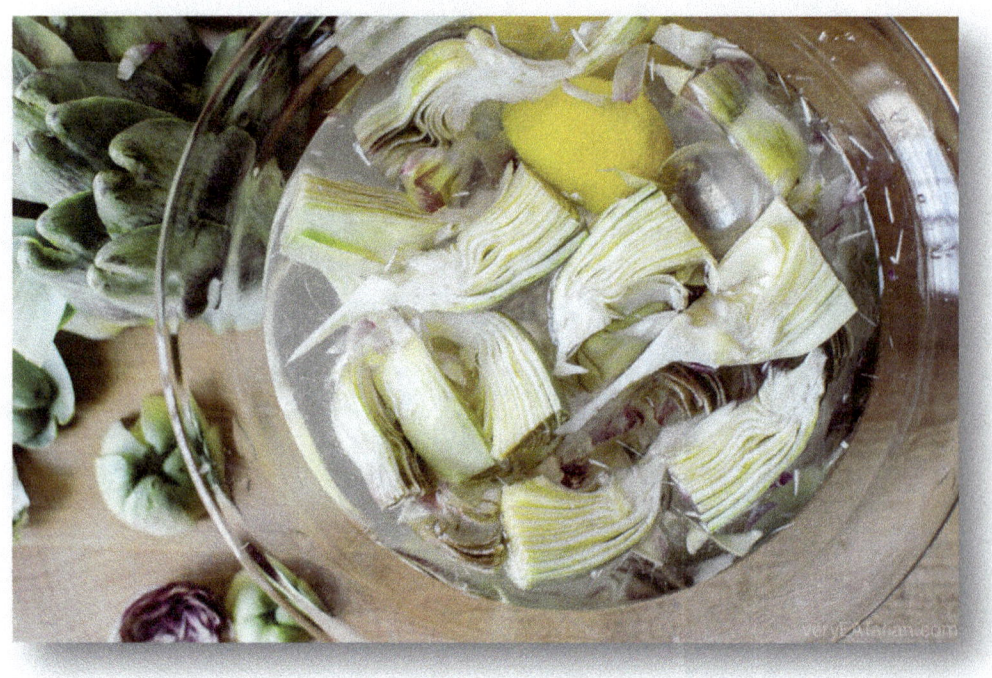

Preparation time: 10 minutes
Cooking time: 12-18 minutes
Servings: 4

Ingredients:

- 6 artichokes
- Olive oil
- 1 tablet of vegetable broth
- Parsley finely cut
- Pepper
- Juice and leftovers of 1 lemon

Directions:

Remove the first layers of the artichoke and garnish with lemon. Grease the mould of the Air Fryer and place the artichokes. Bathe with oil, lemon juice, and the shredded pill. Schedule at 180°C for 12-18 minutes. Serve up hot.

Nutrition:

Energy (calories): 121 kcal
Protein: 8.21 g
Fat: 0.42 g
Carbohydrates: 27.43 g

Orange Lava Cake

Preparation time: 10 minutes
Cooking time: 20 minutes
Servings: 3

Ingredients:
- One tbsp. flax meal combined with two tbsp. water
- Four tbsp. coconut sugar
- Two tbsp. olive oil
- Four tbsp. almond milk
- Four tbsp. whole wheat flour
- One tbsp. cocoa powder
- ½ tsp. Baking powder
- ½ tsp. orange zest, grated

Directions:
In a bowl, mix flax meal with sugar, oil, milk, flour, cocoa powder, baking powder and orange zest, stir very well and pour this into a greased ramekin that fits your air fryer.
Add ramekin to your air fryer, cook at 320 degrees F for 20 minutes and serve warm.
Enjoy!

Nutrition:
Calories 191
Fat 7 g

Fiber 8g
Carbs 13g
Protein 4 g

Cinnamon Apples

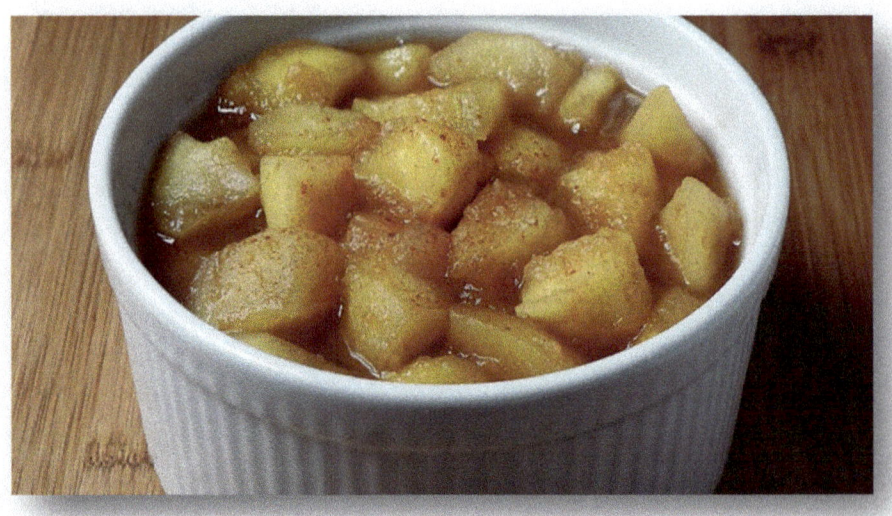

Preparation time: 10 minutes
Cooking time: 10 minutes
Servings: 4

Ingredients:
- Two tsp. cinnamon powder
- Five apples, cored and cut into chunks
- ½ tsp. nutmeg powder
- One tbsp. maple syrup
- ½ cup of water
- Four tbsp. vegetable oil

- ¼ cup whole wheat flour
- ¾ cup old-fashioned rolled oats
- ¼ cup of coconut sugar

Directions:

Put the apples in a pan that fits your air fryer, add cinnamon, nutmeg, maple syrup and water.

Add oil mixed with oats, sugar and flour, stir, spread on top of the apples, introduce in your air fryer, cook at 350 degrees F for 10 minutes and serve them warm.

Enjoy!

Nutrition:

Calories 180

Fat 6g

Fiber 8g

Carbs 19g

Protein 12g

Carrot and Pineapple Cinnamon Bread

Preparation time: 10 minutes
Cooking time: 45 minutes
Servings: 6

Ingredients:
- 5 ounces whole wheat flour
- ¾ tsp. baking powder
- ½ tsp. baking soda
- ½ tsp. cinnamon powder
- ¼ tsp. nutmeg, ground
- One tbsp. flax meal combined with two tbsp. water
- Three tbsp. coconut cream
- ½ cup of sugar
- ¼ cup pineapple juice
- Four tbsp. sunflower oil
- 1/3 cup carrots, grated
- 1/3 cup pecans, toasted and chopped
- 1/3 cup coconut flakes, shredded
- Cooking spray

Directions:
In a bowl, mix flour with baking soda and powder, salt, cinnamon, nutmeg, and stir.

In another bowl, mix the flax meal with coconut cream, sugar, pineapple juice, oil, carrots, pecans and coconut flakes and stir well.

Put together the two mixtures and stir well until combined, pour into a springform pan greased with cooking spray, move to your air fryer and cook at 320 degrees F for 45 minutes.

Leave the cake to cool down, cut and serve it.

Enjoy!

Nutrition:

Calories 180

Fat 6g

Fiber 2g

Carbs 12g

Protein 4 g

Cocoa and Coconut Bars

Preparation time: 10 minutes
Cooking time: 14 minutes
Servings: 12

Ingredients:
- 6 ounces coconut oil, melted
- Three tbsp. Flax meal combined with three tbsp. water
- 3 ounces of cocoa powder
- Two tsp. vanilla
- ½ tsp. baking powder
- 4 ounces coconut cream
- Five tbsp. coconut sugar

Directions:

In a blender, mix the flax meal with oil, cocoa powder, baking powder, vanilla, cream and sugar and pulse.

Pour this into a lined baking dish that fits your air fryer, introduce in the fryer at 320 degrees F, bake for 14 minutes, slice into rectangles and serve.

Enjoy!

Nutrition:

Calories 178

Fat 14g

Fiber 2g

Carbs 12g

Protein 5 g

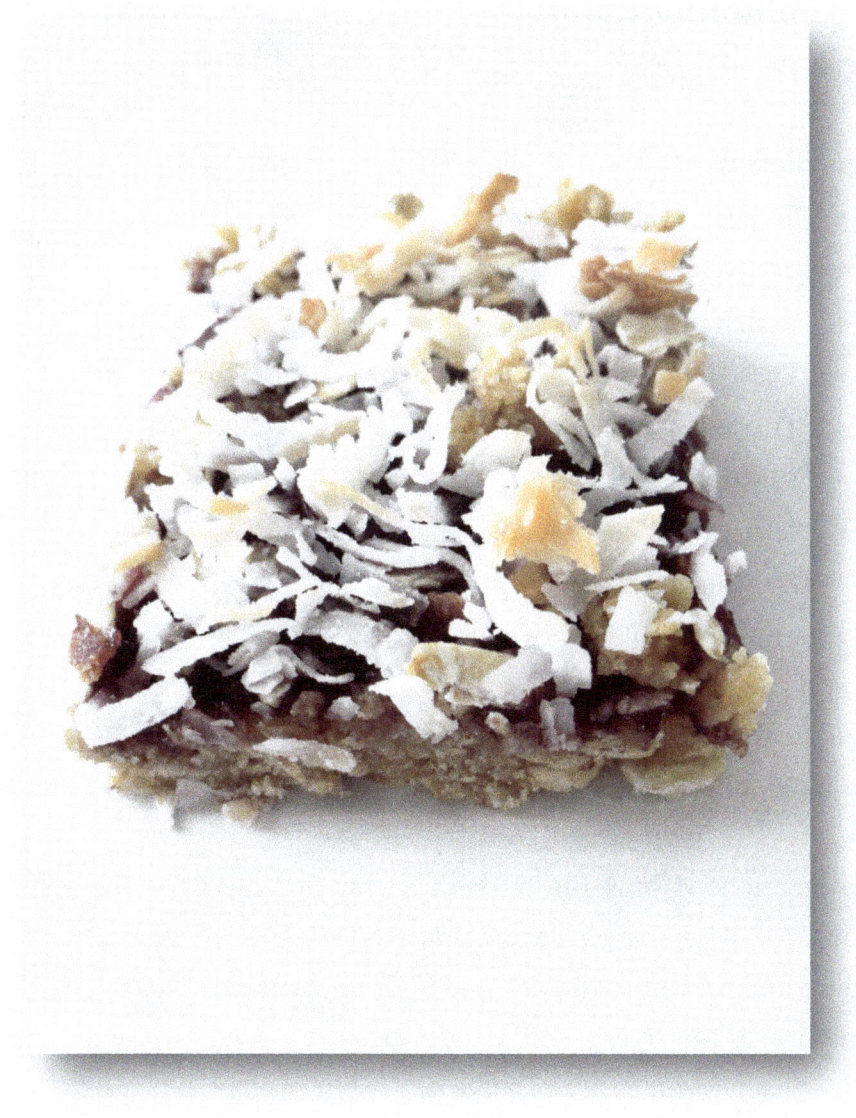

Vanilla Cake

Preparation time: 10 minutes
Cooking time: 25 minutes
Servings: 12

Ingredients:
- Six tbsp. black tea powder
- 2 cups almond milk, heated
- 2 cups of coconut sugar
- Three tbsp. Flax meal combined with three tbsp. water
- Two tsp. vanilla extract
- ½ cup of vegetable oil
- Three and ½ cups whole wheat flour
- One tsp. baking soda
- Three tsp. baking powder

Directions:

In a bowl, mix heated milk with tea powder, stir and leave aside for now.

In a larger bowl, mix the oil with sugar, flax meal, vanilla extract, baking powder, baking soda and flour and stir everything well.

Add tea and milk mix, stir well and pour into a greased cake pan.

Introduce in the fryer, cook at 330 degrees F for 25 minutes, leave aside to cool down, slice and serve it.

Enjoy!

Nutrition:

Calories 180

Fat 4g

Fiber 4g

Carbs 6g

Protein 2g

Sweet Apple Cupcakes

Preparation time: 10 minutes
Cooking time: 20 minutes
Servings: 4

Ingredients:
- Four tbsp. vegetable oil
- Three tbsp. Flax meal combined with three tbsp. water
- ½ cup pure applesauce
- Two tsp. cinnamon powder
- One tsp. vanilla extract
- One apple, cored and chopped
- Four tsp. maple syrup
- ¾ cup whole wheat flour
- ½ tsp. baking powder

Directions:

Heat a pan put the vegetable oil over medium heat, add applesauce, vanilla, flax meal, maple syrup, stir, take off the heat and cool down.

Add flour, cinnamon, baking powder and apples, whisk, pour into a cupcake pan, introduce in your air fryer at 350 degrees F and bake for 20 minutes.

Transfer cupcakes to a platter and serve them warm.

Enjoy!

Nutrition:

Calories 200

Fat 3g

Fiber 1g

Carbs 5g

Protein 4g

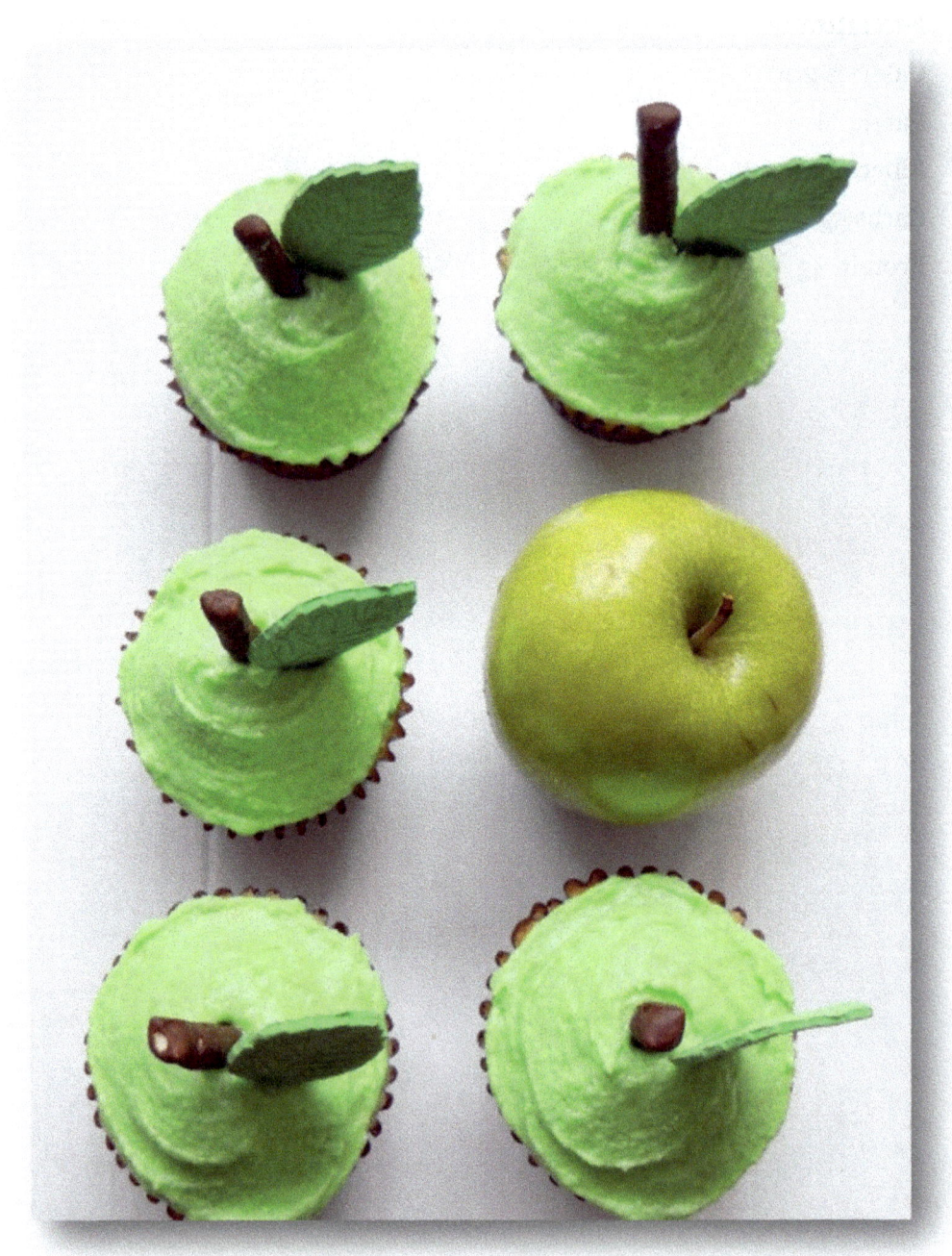

Orange Bread with Almonds

Preparation time: 20 minutes
Cooking time: 40 minutes
Servings: 8

Ingredients:
- One orange, peeled and sliced
- Juice of 2 oranges
- Three tbsp. vegetable oil
- Two tbsp. flax meal combined with two tbsp. water
- ¾ cup coconut sugar+ 2 tbsp.
- ¾ cup whole wheat flour
- ¾ cup almonds, ground

Directions:
Grease a loaf pan with some oil, sprinkle two tbsp. of sugar and arrange orange slices on the bottom.
In a bowl, mix the oil with ¾ cup sugar, almonds, flour and orange juice, stir, spoon this over orange slices, place the pan in your air fryer and cook at 360 degrees F for 40 minutes.
Slice and serve the bread right away.
Enjoy!

Nutrition:
Calories 202
Fat 3g

Fiber 2g
Carbs 6g
Protein 6g

Tangerine Cake

Preparation time: 10 minutes
Cooking time: 20 minutes
Servings: 8

Ingredients:
- ¾ cup of coconut sugar
- 2 cups whole wheat flour
- ¼ cup olive oil
- ½ cup almond milk
- One tsp. cider vinegar
- ½ tsp. vanilla extract
- Juice and zest of 2 lemons
- Juice and zest of 1 tangerine

Directions:
In a prepared bowl, mix flour with sugar and stir.
In another bowl, mix oil with milk, vinegar, vanilla extract, lemon juice and zest, tangerine zest and flour, whisk very well, pour this into a cake pan that fits your air fryer, introduce in the fryer and cook at 360 degrees F for 20 minutes.
Serve right away.
Enjoy!

Nutrition:

Calories 210

Fat 1g

Fiber 1g

Carbs 6g

Protein 4g

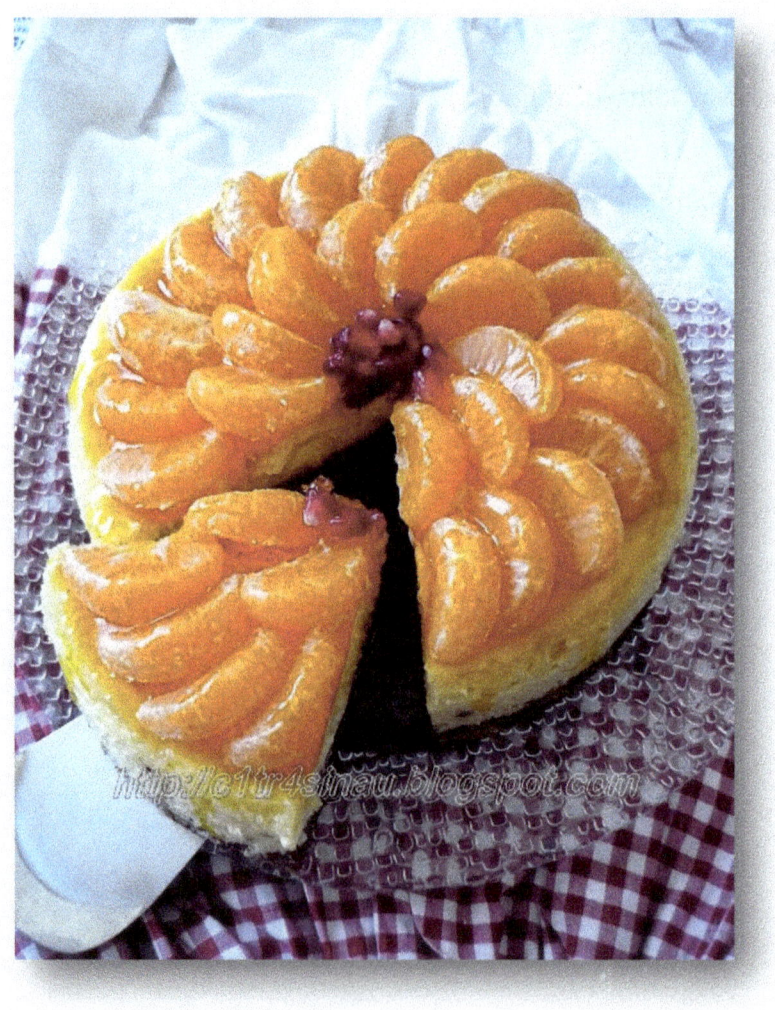

Maple Tomato Bread

Preparation time: 10 minutes
Cooking time: 30 minutes
Servings: 4
Ingredients:
- One and ½ cups whole wheat flour
- One tsp. cinnamon powder
- One tsp. baking powder
- One tsp. baking soda
- ¾ cup maple syrup
- 1 cup tomatoes, chopped
- ½ cup olive oil
- Two tbsp. apple cider vinegar

Directions:

In a bowl, mix flour with baking powder, baking soda, cinnamon and maple syrup and stir well.

In another bowl, mix tomatoes with olive oil and vinegar and stir well.

Combine the two mixtures, stir well, pour into a greased loaf pan that fits your air fryer, introduce in the fryer and cook at 360 degrees F for 30 minutes.

Leave the cake to cool down, slice and serve.

Enjoy!

Nutrition:

Calories 203

Fat 2g

Fiber 1g

Carbs 12g

Protein 4 g

Lemon Squares

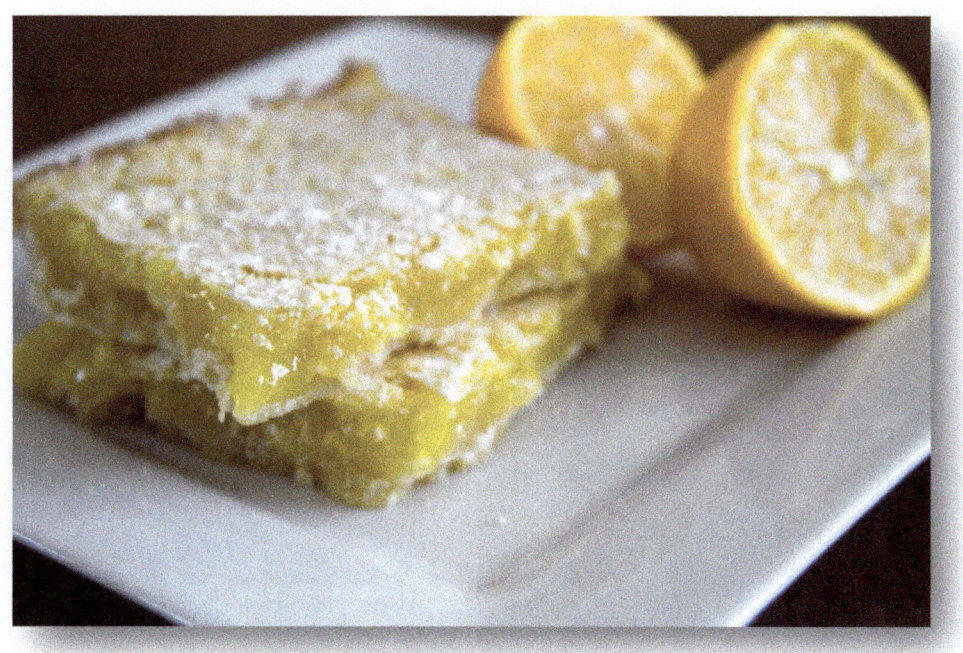

Preparation time: 10 minutes
Cooking time: 30 minutes
Servings: 6

Ingredients:
- 1 cup whole wheat flour
- ½ cup of vegetable oil
- One and ¼ cups of coconut sugar

- One medium banana
- Two tsp. lemon peel, grated
- Two tbsp. lemon juice
- Two tbsp. Flax meal combined with two tbsp. water
- ½ tsp. baking powder

Directions:

In a bowl, mix flour with ¼ cup sugar and oil, stir well, press on the bottom of a pan that fits your air fryer, introduce in the fryer and bake at 350 degrees F for 14 minutes.

In another prepared bowl, mix the rest of the sugar with lemon juice, lemon peel, banana, baking powder, stir using your mixer and spread over baked crust.

Bake for 15 minutes more, leave aside to cool down, cut into medium squares and serve cold.

Enjoy!

Nutrition:

Calories 140

Fat 4g

Fibre 1g

Carbs 12g

Protein 1g

Dates and Cashew Sticks

Preparation time: 10 minutes
Cooking time: 15 minutes
Servings: 6

Ingredients:
- 1/3 cup stevia
- ¼ cup almond meal
- One tbsp. almond butter
- One and ½ cups cashews, chopped
- Four dates, chopped
- ¾ cup coconut, shredded
- One tbsp. chia seeds

Directions:
In a bowl, mix stevia with almond meal, almond butter, cashews, coconut, dates and chia seeds and stir well again.
Spread this on a lined baking sheet that fits your air fryer, press well, introduce in the fryer and cook at 300 degrees F for 15 minutes .
Leave the mix to cool down, cut into medium sticks and serve.
Enjoy!

Nutrition:
Calories 162
Fat 4g
Fibre 7g

Carbs 5g
Protein 6g

Grape Pudding

Preparation time: 10 minutes
Cooking time: 40 minutes
Servings: 6

Ingredients:
- 1 cup grapes curd
- 3 cups grapes
- Three and ½ ounces maple syrup
- Three tbsp. Flax meal combined with three tbsp. water
- 2 ounces coconut butter, melted
- Three and ½ ounces of almond milk
- ½ cup almond flour
- ½ tsp. baking powder

Directions:

In a bowl, mix half of the fruit curd with the grapes, stir and divide into six heatproof ramekins.

In a prepared bowl, mix the flax meal with maple syrup, melted coconut butter, the rest of the curd, baking powder, milk and flour and stir well.

Divide this into the ramekins and introduce in the fryer and cook at 200 degrees F for 40 minutes.

Leave puddings to cool down and serve!

Enjoy!

Nutrition:

Calories 230

Fat 22g

Fibre 3g

Carbs 17g

Protein 8 g

Coconut and Pumpkin Seeds Bars

Preparation time: 10 minutes
Cooking time: 35 minutes
Servings: 4

Ingredients:

- 1 cup coconut, shredded
- ½ cup almonds
- ½ cup pecans, chopped
- Two tbsp. coconut sugar
- ½ cup pumpkin seeds
- ½ cup sunflower seeds
- Two tbsp. sunflower oil
- One tsp. nutmeg, ground
- One tsp. pumpkin pie spice

Directions:

In a bowl, mix almonds and pecans with pumpkin seeds, sunflower seeds, coconut, nutmeg and pie spice and stir well.

Heat a pan put the sunflower oil over medium heat, add sugar, stir well, pour this over nuts and coconut mix and stir well.

Spread this on a lined baking sheet that fits your air fryer, introduce in your air fryer and cook at 300 degrees F and bake for 25 minutes.

Leave the mix aside to cool down, cut and serve.

Enjoy!

Nutrition:
Calories 252
Fat 7g
Fibre 8g
Carbs 12g
Protein 7g

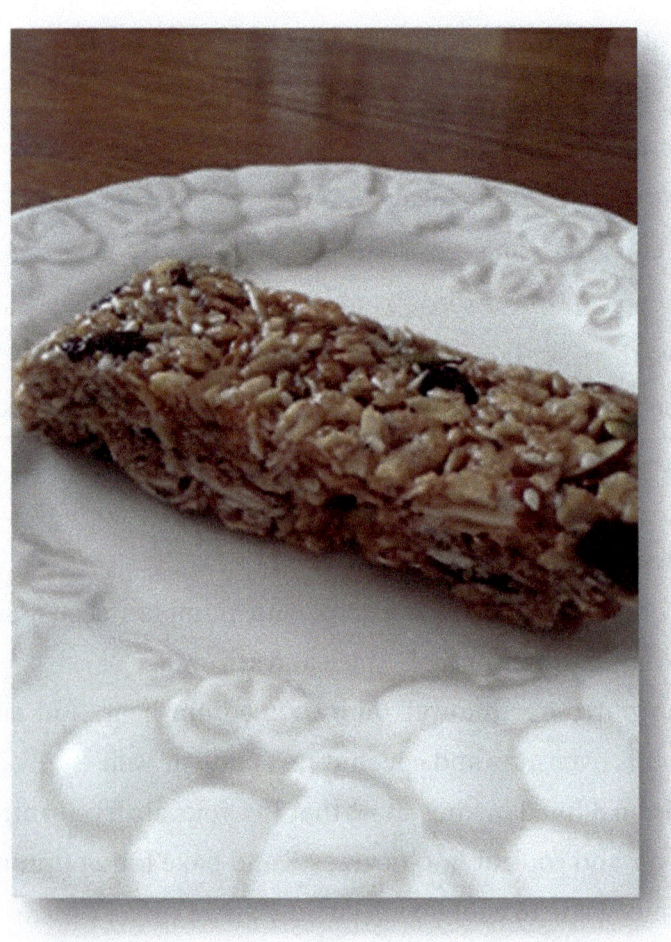

Cinnamon Bananas

Preparation time: 10 minutes
Cooking time: 15 minutes
Servings: 4

Ingredients:
- Three tbsp. coconut butter
- Two tbsp. flax meal combined with two tbsp. water
- Eight bananas, peeled and halved
- ½ cup of cornflour
- Three tbsp. cinnamon powder
- 1 cup vegan breadcrumb s

Directions:

Heat a pan with the butter over medium-high heat, add breadcrumbs, stir and cook for 4 minutes and then transfer to a bowl.
Roll each banana in flour, flax meal and breadcrumbs mix.
Arrange bananas in your air fryer's basket, dust with cinnamon sugar and cook at 280 degrees F for 10 minutes.
Transfer to plates and serve.
Enjoy!

Nutrition:
Calories 214
Fat 1g
Fibre 4g

Carbs 12g
Protein 4 g

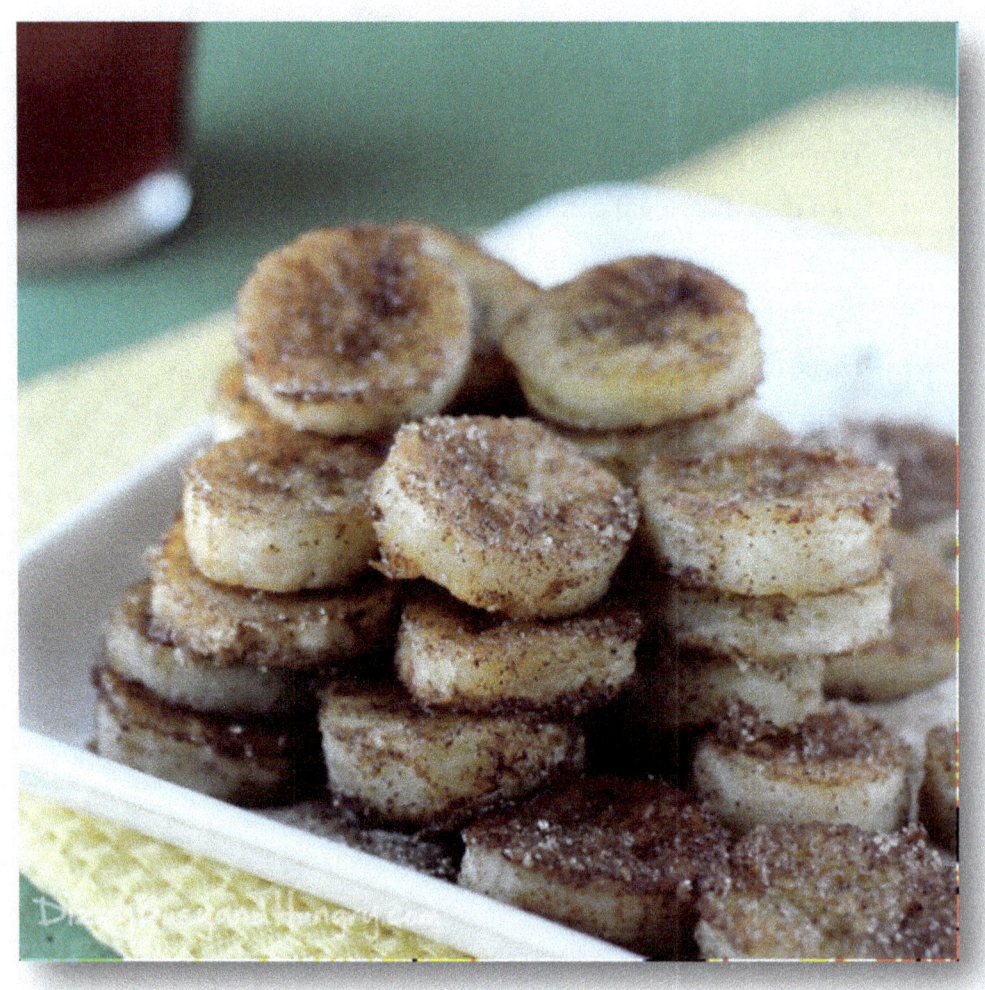

Coffee Pudding

Preparation time: 10 minutes
Cooking time: 10 minutes
Servings: 4

Ingredients:
- 4 ounces coconut butter
- 4 ounces dark vegan chocolate, chopped
- Juice of ½ orange
- One tsp. baking powder
- 2 ounces whole wheat flour
- ½ tsp. instant coffee
- Two tbsp. Flax meal combined with two tbsp. water
- 2 ounces of coconut sugar

Directions:
Heat a pan with the coconut butter over medium heat, add chocolate and orange juice, stir well and take off the heat.
In a bowl, mix sugar with instant coffee and flax meal, beat using your mixer, add chocolate mix, flour, salt, baking powder, and stir well.
Pour this into a greased pan, introduce in your air fryer, cook at 360 degrees F for about 10 minutes, divide between plates and serve.
Enjoy!

Nutrition:

Calories 189

Fat 6g

Fibre 4g

Carbs 14g

Protein 3 g

Blueberry Cake

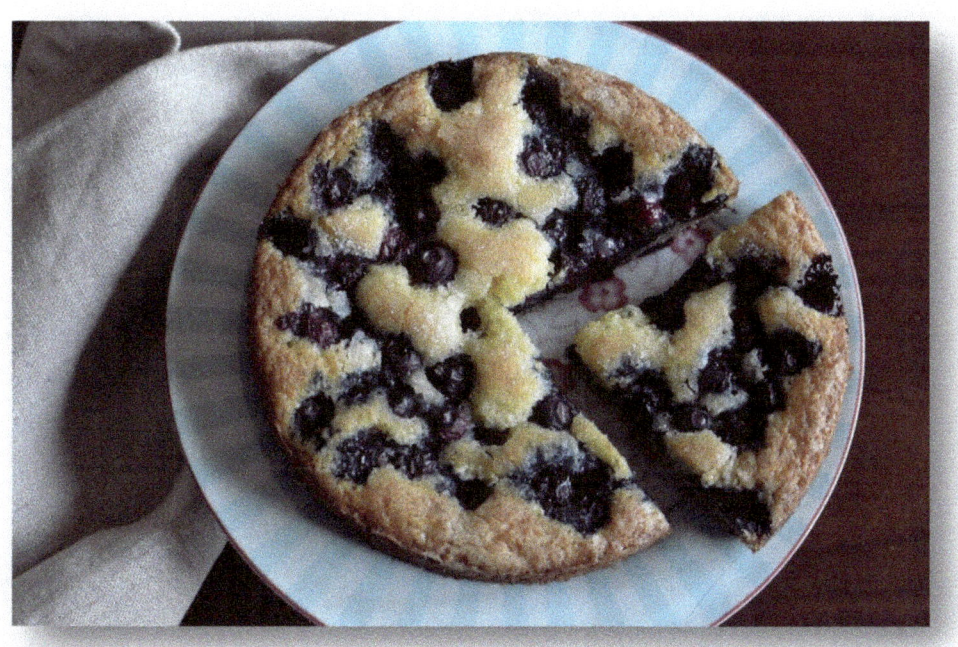

Preparation time: 10 minutes
Cooking time: 30 minutes
Servings: 6

Ingredients:
- ½ cup whole wheat flour
- ¼ tsp. baking powder
- ¼ tsp. stevia
- ¼ cup blueberries
- 1/3 cup almond milk

- One tsp. olive oil
- One tsp. flaxseed, ground
- ½ tsp. lemon zest, grated
- ¼ tsp. vanilla extract
- ¼ tsp. lemon extract
- Cooking spray

Directions:

In a bowl, mix flour with baking powder, stevia, blueberries, milk, oil, flaxseeds, lemon zest, vanilla extract and lemon extract and whisk well.

Spray a cake pan with cooking spray, line it with parchment paper, pour cake batter, introduce in the fryer and cook at 350 degrees F for 30 minutes.

Leave the cake to cool down, slice and serve.

Enjoy!

Nutrition:

Calories 210

Fat 4g

Fibre 4g

Carbs 10g

Protein 4g

Peach Cinnamon Cobbler

Preparation time: 10 minutes
Cooking time: 30 minutes
Servings: 4

Ingredients:
- 4 cups peaches, peeled and sliced
- ¼ cup of coconut suga r
- ½ tsp. cinnamon powder
- One and ½ cups vegan crackers, crushed
- ¼ cup stevia
- ¼ tsp. nutmeg, ground
- ½ cup almond milk
- One tsp. vanilla extract
- Cooking spray

Directions:
In a bowl, mix peaches with coconut sugar and cinnamon and stir.
In a separate bowl, mix crackers with stevia, nutmeg, almond milk and vanilla extract and stir.
Spray a pie pan that fits your air fryer with cooking spray and spread peaches on the bottom.
Add crackers mix, spread, introduce into the fryer and cook at 350 degrees F for 30 minutes
Divide the cobbler between plates and serve.
Enjoy!

Nutrition:

Calories 201

Fat 4g

Fibre 4g

Carbs 7g

Protein 3g

Vegan Fruits

Caramelized Bananas

Preparation time: 10 minutes

Cooking time: 60 minutes

Servings: 2

Ingredients:
- Ripe bananas.
- ½ cup of maple syrup
- Cinnamon powder
- A little water

Directions:

Cut the peeled banana into pieces. Place them in a small pot with a little olive oil and sprinkle with the ingredient—Fry in Air Fryer for 58 minutes at 180°C. Serve up with bread, rice or vegetables.

Nutrition:

Energy (calories): 378 kcal

Protein: 1.98 g

Fat: 0.95 g

Carbohydrates: 96.93 g

Banana Rolls

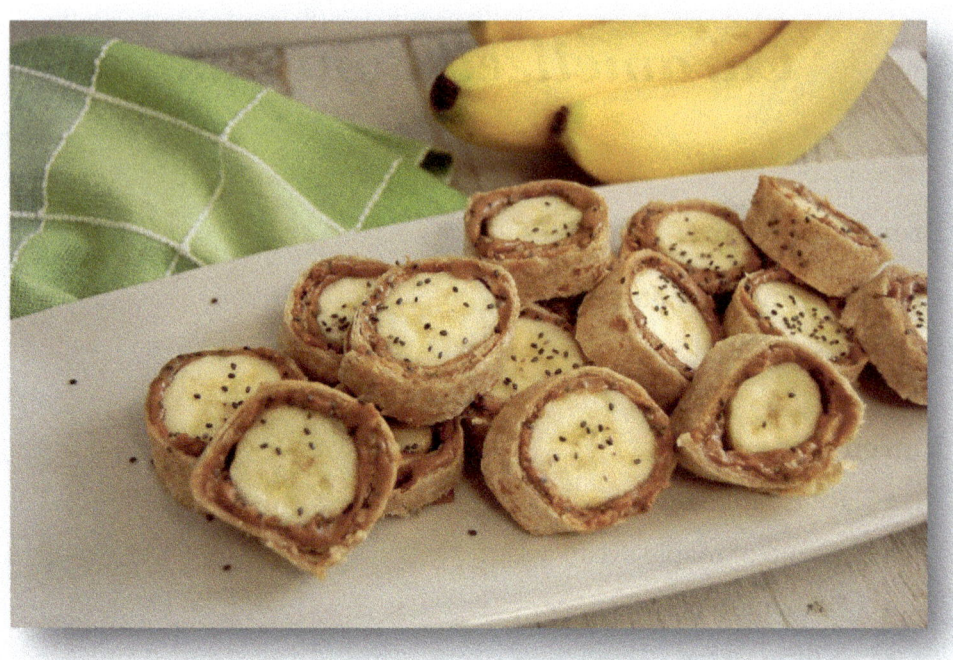

Preparation time: 10 minutes
Cooking time: 60 minutes
Servings: 4

Ingredients:
- 3 ripe bananas
- Optional English sauce
- Agaragar prepared in water
- Wheat flour
- 1 onion

- 200gr of soy meat
- Olives
- Sweet pepper
- Garlic
- Dressing

Directions:

Hydrate the meat for 10 minutes. Drain very well. Peel and chop the bananas in half in two slices each. To part, marinate the meat and fry with the garlic. Add the other minced Ingredients to the meat. Form circles with the pieces and fix them with the chopsticks. Fill with the meat; let it rest a little so that the liquid comes out. Seal with egg and a little wheat flour. Place in the Air Fryer for 48 minutes at 180°C. Watch the cooking. Turn, so it cooks evenly.

Nutrition:

Energy (calories): 53 kcal
Protein: 5.3 g
Fat: 0.38 g
Carbohydrates: 8.33 g

Fried Omelet of Ripe Bananas

Preparation time: 10 minutes
Cooking time: 8-12 minutes
Servings: 6

Ingredients:
- 6 Ripe bananas
- 1 Cup of wheat
- Grated vegan hard cheese
- Sugar
- Cinnamon

Directions:

Process or grind bananas and knead with flour and cheese to taste. Add sugar and cinnamon powder to taste. Knead very well and shape with your hand—Fry in Air Fryer for 8-12 minutes at 180°C. Halfway through the cooking, turn around to cook on both sides.

Nutrition:
Energy (calories): 68 kcal
Protein: 2.64 g
Fat: 0.5 g
Carbohydrates: 14.39 g

Sweet Corn Pies

Preparation time: 10 minutes
Cooking time: 6-10 minutes
Servings: 2

Ingredients:
- 1 ¼ cup of bread flour
- ¾ cup of water.
- ½ cup of shredded or molasses paper
- 2 tsp. of sweet anise
- ½ tsp. of salt

Directions:

Place the flour, put water, and salt in a bowl. Mix well until the dough is compact. Little by little, the paper and anise are added. Knead well, and 12 balls are formed. It is a shaped, thin corn cake. Fry in Air Fryer for 6-10 minutes at 160°C. They eat with coffee, tea, alone or to taste.

Nutrition:

Energy (calories): 561 kcal
Protein: 10.63 g
Fat: 1.84 g
Carbohydrates: 126.13 g

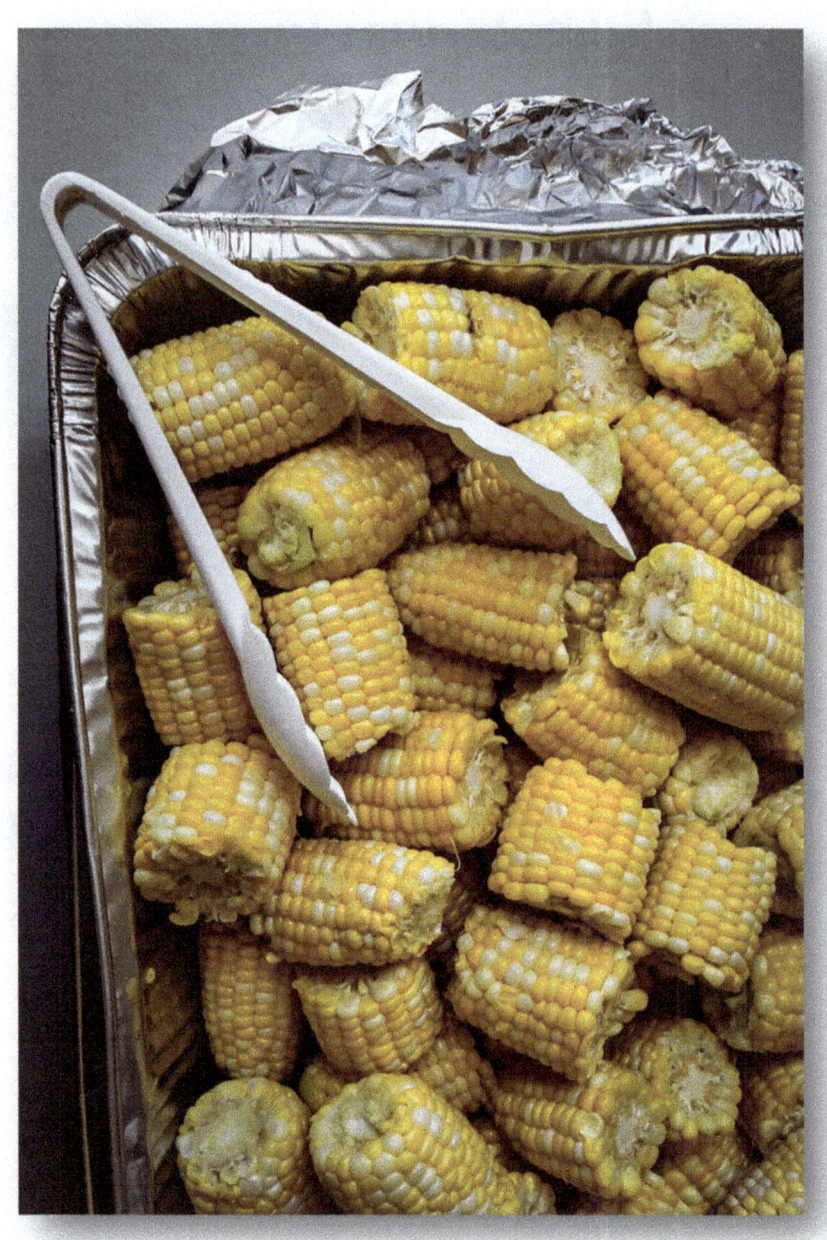

Banana Pie

Preparation time: 10 minutes
Cooking time: 5-10 minutes
Servings: 3

Ingredients:
- 3 Ripe bananas
- 1/2 cup flour
- Beans
- Red pepper
- Onion
- Coriander
- Oil
- Water
- Salt

Directions:
For the filling, prepare a pot with beans, red pepper, onion, coriander and some spices. In a pot of water with sugar, cook the bananas peeled and cut into cubes. When softened, remove and ultimately crush the bananas. Mix with the flour. Form some balls with the dough and mash them well. Place a portion of the filling in the center and close the tortilla. Seal the pie with your hands and place it in the Air Fryer. Fry for 5 -10 minutes at 180ºC. Serve up.

Nutrition:

Energy (calories): 97 kcal

Protein: 2.86 g

Fat: 0.32 g

Carbohydrates: 20.73 g

Apple Fritters

Preparation time: 10 minutes
Cooking time: 10-15 minutes
Servings: 2

Ingredients:
- 2 large apples
- 200 grams of flour
- Salt
- A ¼ liter of cider or beer
- 1 tsp. olive oil
- Sugar

Directions:
First, peel the apples and remove the seeds. Cut into rings and sprinkle sugar. Add the flour to a bowl and add salt, oil, and beer. Mix. Sprinkle the apples in the mixture and place them in the Air Fryer tray with butter paper. Fry for 10 -15 minutes at 180ºC. Add sugar and Serve up hot.

Nutrition:
Energy (calories): 500 kcal
Protein: 10.91 g
Fat: 3.61 g
Carbohydrates: 107.11 g

Fried Apples

Preparation time: 5 minutes
Cooking time: 6 minutes
Servings: 2

Ingredients:
- 2 apples
- 2/3 cups cornstarch
- 1 spoon of sugar
- 1/8 tsp. of cinnamon
- ½ cup of caramel sauce

Directions:

Peel and cut the apples. Mix with the cornstarch. Fry in the Air Fryer for 6 minutes at 180°C. Flip to be cooked on both sides. Spray cinnamon and sugar when serving.

Nutrition:

Energy (calories): 277 kcal
Protein: 1.59 g
3%
Fat: 0.44 g
Carbohydrates: 68.78 g

Banana Salad

Preparation time: 10 minutes
Cooking time: 6-10 minutes
Servings: 2

Ingredients:

- 2 large green bananas cut into squares
- 8 sweet peppers cut in squares
- 1 hot pepper
- ½ cup fresh cut coriander
- The juice of 5 lemon
- ½ cup of olive oil
- 1 tsp. salt
- 2 cloves garlic crushed
- Pepper

Directions:

In the Air Fryer mould, place the bananas with salt and the juice of 1 lemon. Cover and program it at 140°C for 6 -10 minutes. Take out and let cool. Mix in a salad bowl the cooked bananas, chilli, coriander and spicy to your taste. In another bowl, mix the juice of 4 lemons, garlic, oil, salt and pepper to taste. Add to the previously made salad and Serve up fresh, or Reserve up in the fridge.

Nutrition:

Energy (calories): 695 kcal

Protein: 6.37 g

Fat: 55.13 g

Carbohydrates: 55.45 g

Salad of Rice and Avocados

Preparation time: 10 minutes
Cooking time: 10-15 minutes
Servings: 4

Ingredients:
- 2 avocados in slices
- 1 cup of rice
- 1 can of drained peas
- 2 spring onions julienne
- 1 cucumbe r
- 1 tablet of vegetable broth
- 1 carrot in small cubes
- Stuffed Olives
- Olive oil
- Lemon juice
- Salt, pepper, and water

Directions:

In the mould of the Air Fryer, add the rice, a little oil, and salt. Mix and program it at 180°C for 10- 15 minutes. Let cool. Mix pepper, oil, lemon juice and the shredded pill. Mix all together all the Ingredients with the rice and add the vinaigrette. Serve up fresh.

Nutrition:

Energy (calories): 276 kcal

Protein: 6.74 g

Fat: 21.18 g

Carbohydrates: 28.1 g

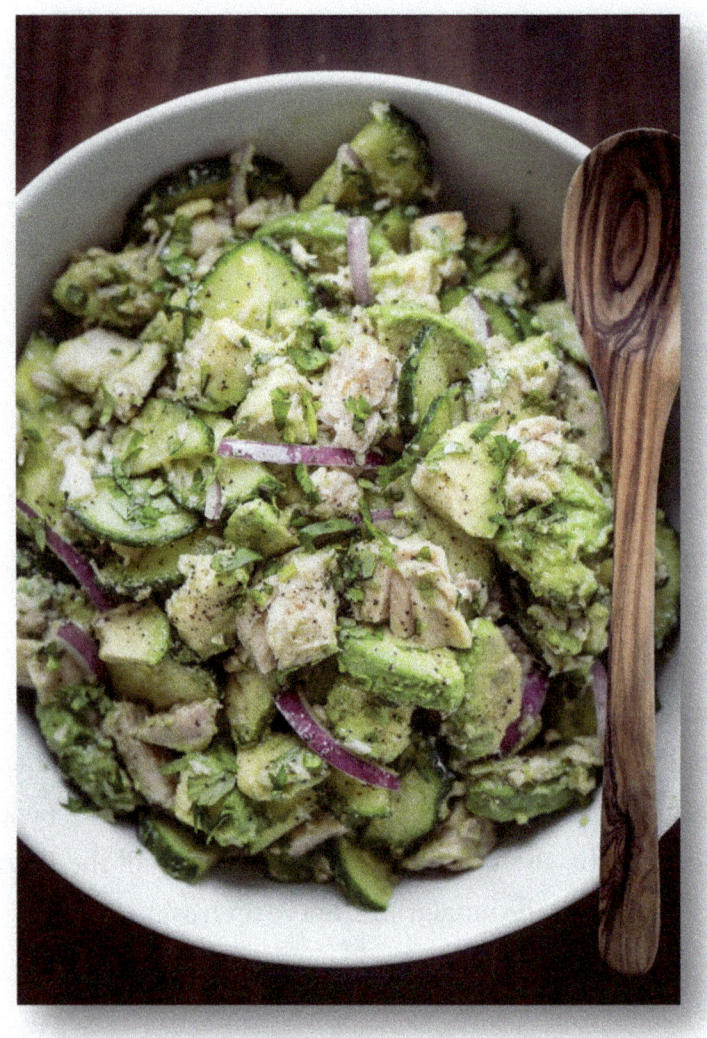

Vegan Dessert

Tomato Cake

Preparation time: 10 minutes
Cooking time: 30 minutes
Servings: 4

Ingredients:
One and ½ cups flour
1 tsp. cinnamon powder
1 tsp. baking powder
1 tsp. baking soda
¾ cup maple syrup
1 cup tomatoes chopped
½ cup olive oil
2 tbsp. apple cider vinegar

Directions:
In a bowl, mix flour with baking powder, baking soda, cinnamon and maple syrup and stir well.
In another bowl, mix tomatoes with olive oil and vinegar and stir well.
Combine the two mixtures, stir well, pour into a greased round pan that fits your air fryer, introduce in the fryer and cook at 360 degrees F for 30 minutes.
Leave the cake to cool down, slice and serve.

Enjoy!

Nutrition:
Calories 153
Fat 2g
Fibre 1g
Carbs 25g
Protein 4 g

Berries Mix

Preparation time: 5 minutes
Cooking time: 6 minutes
Servings: 4

Ingredients:
- 2 tbsp. lemon juice
- One and ½ tbsp. maple syrup
- One and ½ tbsp. champagne vinegar
- One tbsp. olive oil
- 1 pound strawberries, halved
- One and ½ cups blueberries
- ¼ cup basil leaves, torn

Directions:
In a pan that fits your air fryer, mix lemon juice with maple syrup and vinegar, bring and let it boil over medium-high heat, add oil, blueberries, strawberries, stir, and introduce in your air fryer and cook at temperature of 310 degrees F for 6 minutes.
Sprinkle basil on top and serve!
Enjoy!

Nutrition:
Calories 163
Fat 4g
Fiber 4g

Carbs 10g
Protein 2.1g

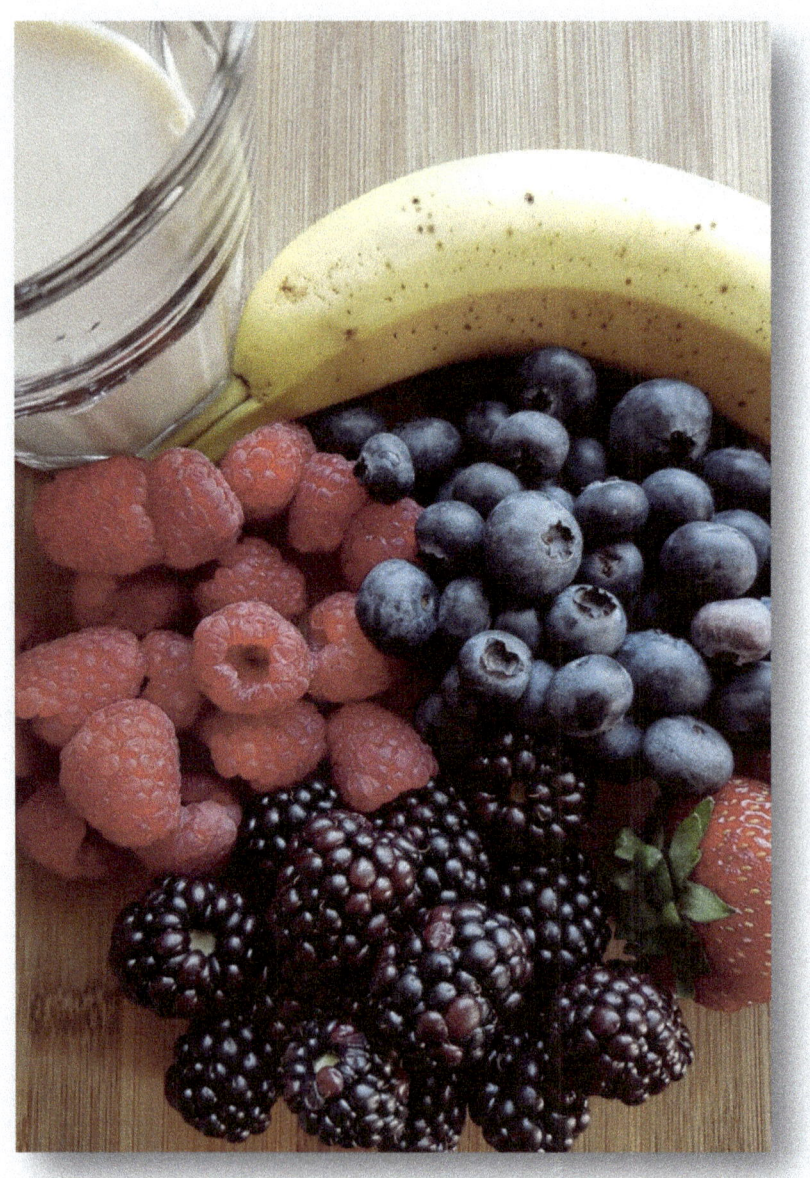

Passion Fruit Pudding

Preparation time: 10 minutes
Cooking time: 40 minutes
Servings: 6

Ingredients:
- 1 cup Paleo passion fruit curd
- Four passion fruits, pulp and seeds
- Three and ½ ounces maple syrup
- ¾ cup of silken tofu
- 2 ounces ghee, melted
- Three and ½ ounces of almond milk
- ½ cup almond flour
- ½ tsp. baking powder

Directions:
In a bowl, mix half of the fruit curd with passion fruit seeds and pulp, stir and divide into six heatproof ramekins.
In a bowl, whisk silken tofu with maple syrup, ghee, the rest of the curd, baking powder, milk and flour and stir well.
Divide this into the ramekins and introduce in the fryer and cook at 200 degrees F for 40 minutes.
Leave puddings to cool down and serve!
Enjoy!

Nutrition:
Calories 430
Fat 22g
Fiber 3g
Carbs 7g
Protein 8g

Pumpkin Cookies

Preparation time: 10 minutes
Cooking time: 15 minutes
Servings: 24

Ingredients:
- Two and ½ cups flour
- ½ tsp. baking soda
- 1 tbsp. flaxseed, ground
- 3 tbsp. water
- ½ cup of pumpkin flesh, mashed
- ¼ cup maple syrup
- 2 tbsp. butter
- 1 tsp. vanilla extract
- ½ cup dark chocolate chips

Directions:
In a bowl, mix flaxseed with water, stir and leave aside for a few minutes.
In another bowl, mix flour with salt and baking soda.
In a third bowl, mix maple syrup with pumpkin puree, butter, vanilla extract and flaxseed.
Combine flour with maple syrup mix and chocolate chips and stir.
Scoop one tbsp. of cookie dough into a lined baking sheet that fits your air fryer, repeat with the rest of the dough, introduce them to your air fryer and cook at 350 degrees F for 15 minutes.

Leave cookies to cool down and serve. Enjoy!

Nutrition:

Calories 140

Fat 2g

Fibre 2g

Carbs 7g

Protein 10g

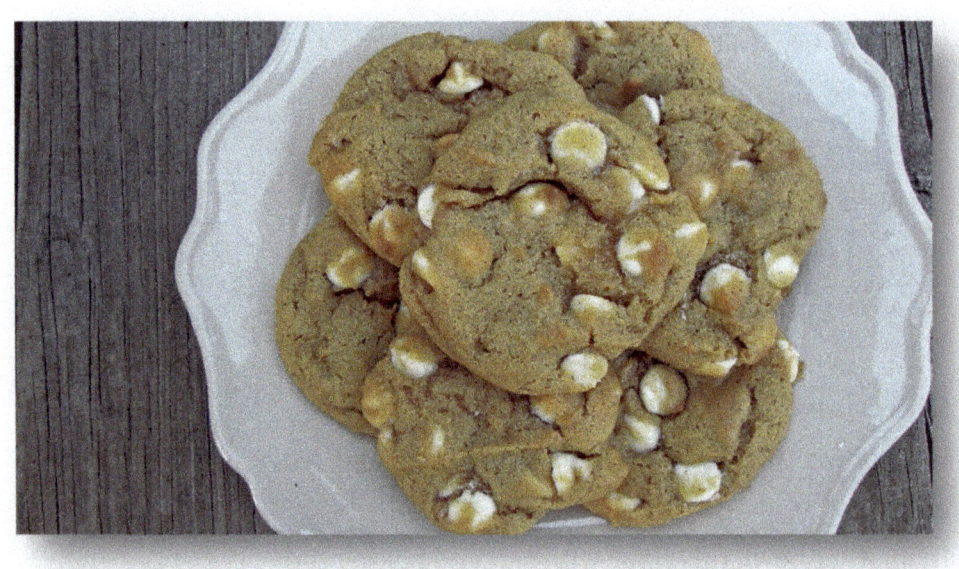

Figs and Coconut Butter Mix

Preparation time: 6 minutes
Cooking time: 4 minutes
Servings: 3

Ingredients:
- 2 tbsp. coconut butter
- 12 figs, halved
- ¼ cup of sugar
- 1 cup almonds, toasted and chopped

Directions:
Put butter in a pan that fits your air fryer and melt over medium-high heat.
Add figs, sugar and almonds, toss, introduce in your air fryer and cook at 300 degrees F for 4 minutes.
Divide into bowls and serve cold.
Enjoy!

Nutrition:
Calories 170
Fat 4g
Fibre 5g
Carbs 7g
Protein 9g

Pears and Espresso Cream

Preparation time: 10 minutes
Cooking time: 30 minutes
Servings: 4

Ingredients:
- Four pears, halved and cored
- 2 tbsp. lemon juice
- 1 tbsp. sugar
- 2 tbsp. water
- 2 tbsp. vegan butter
- For the cream:
- 1 cup vegan whipped cream
- 1 cup vegan cream cheese
- 1/3 cup sugar
- 2 tbsps. espresso, cold

Directions:

In a bowl, mix pears halves with lemon juice, one tbsp. sugar, vegan butter and water, toss well, transfer them to your air fryer and cook at 360 degrees F for 30 minutes.

Meanwhile, in a bowl, mix vegan whipped cream with vegan cream cheese, 1/3 cup sugar and espresso, whisk well and keep in the fridge until pears are done.

Divide pears on plates, top with espresso cream and serve them. Enjoy!

Nutrition:

Calories 211

Fat 5

Fibre 7

Carbs 8

Protein 7

Chocolate Chip Cookies

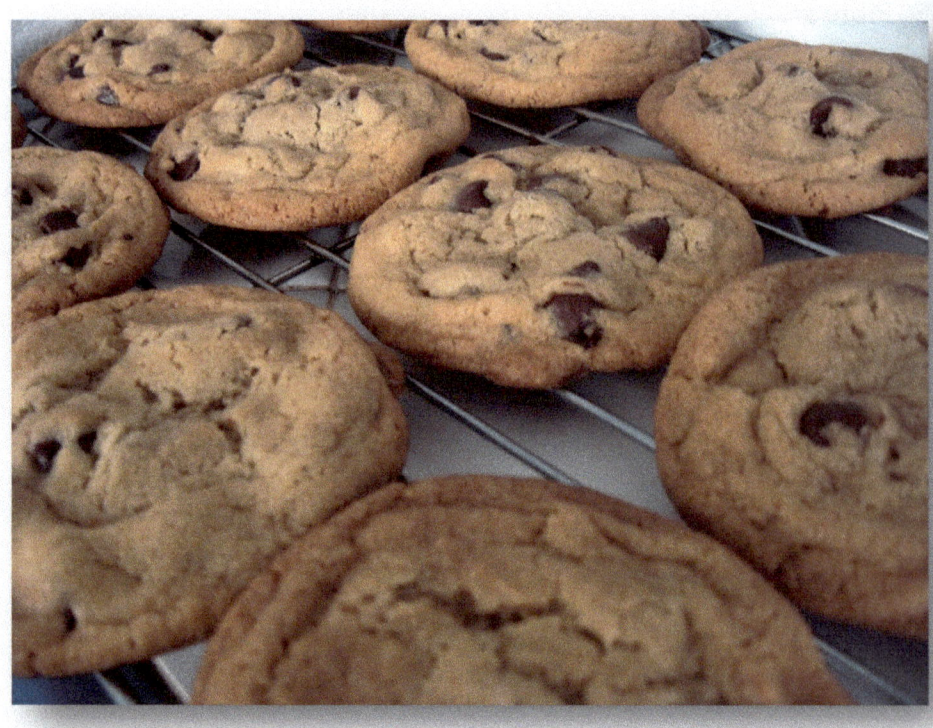

Preparation time: 10 minutes
Cooking time: 7 minutes
Servings: 6 cookies
Bake: 347°F

Ingredients:
- 1 tbsp. refined coconut oil, melted
- 1 tbsp. maple syrup
- 1 tbsp. Nondairy milk
- ½ tsp. vanilla
- ¼ cup plus 2 tbsp. whole-wheat pastry flour or all-purpose gluten-free flour
- 2 tbsp. Coconut sugar
- ¼ tsp. sea salt
- ¼ tsp. baking powder
- 2 tbsps. vegan chocolate chips
- Cooking oil spray this can be (sunflower, safflower, or refined coconut)

Directions:

In a medium bowl, stir together the oil, maple syrup, milk, and vanilla. Add the flour, coconut sugar, salt, and baking powder. Stir just until thoroughly combined. Stir in the chocolate chips.

Preheat the air fryer basket (with a 6-inch round, 2-inch deep baking pan inside) for 2 minutes. Then, spray the pan lightly with oil. Drop a tbsp.ful of the batter onto the pan, leaving a little room in between in case they spread out a bit—Bake for 7 minutes, or until lightly browned. Be careful not to overcook.

Gently transfer to a cooling rack (or plate). Repeat as desired, making all of the cookies at once, or keeping the batter on hand in the fridge to be used later (it will keep refrigerated in an airtight container for about a week). Enjoy warm if possible!

Cooking Tip: These are my "safe" chocolate chip cookies because even if I eat the whole batch over a day or two, I don't feel too horrible about it. Of course, if you have tons of self-control around warm, gooey cookies (are you even human?), feel free to make it double or triple the batch. However, I enjoy keeping the batter on hand in the fridge to make up just a few when I need cookie love.

Nutrition:
Calories: 71
Total fat: 3g
Cholesterol: 0mg
Carbohydrates: 11 g
Fibre: 1g
Protein: 1g

Oatmeal Raisin Cookies

Preparation time: 10 minutes
Cooking time: 7 minutes
Servings: 18 cookies
Bake: 347°F

Ingredients:

- ¼ cup plus ½ tbsp. vegan margarine
- 2½ tbsp. non-dairy milk, plain and unsweetened
- ½ cup of organic sugar
- ½ tsp. vanilla extract
- ½ tsp. plus 1/8 tsp. ground cinnamon
- ½ cup plus two tbsp. flour (whole-wheat pastry, gluten-free all-purpose, or all-purpose)
- ¼ tsp. of sea salt
- ¾ cup rolled oats
- ¼ tsp. baking soda
- ¼ tsp. baking powder
- 2 tbsp. raisins
- Cooking oil spray it can be (sunflower, safflower, or refined coconut)

Directions:

In a medium bowl, using an electric beater, whip the margarine until fluffy.

Add in the milk, sugar, and vanilla. Stir or whip with beaters until well combined.

In a prepared separate bowl, add the cinnamon, flour, salt, oats, baking soda, and baking powder and stir well to combine. Add the dry mixture to the wet mixture and mix everything well with a wooden spoon. Stir in the raisins.

Preheat the air fryer basket (with your 6-inch round, 2-inch deep baking pan inside) for 2 minutes. Then, spray the pan lightly with oil. Drop tbsp.fuls of the batter onto the pan, leaving a little room in between each one as they'll probably spread out a bit—Bake for about 7 minutes, or until lightly browned.

Gently transfer to a cooling rack (or plate), being careful to leave the cookies intact. Repeat as desired, making all of the cookies at once, or keeping the batter on hand in the fridge to be used later (it will keep refrigerated in an airtight container for a week to 10 days).

Substitution Tip: You may substitute coconut oil for the margarine if you prefer. However, if you do this, add a pinch more salt, as the oil will be salt-free, unlike margarine. If you use the vegan margarine as directed, keep in mind that the "pure fat" variety will work best (as opposed to the whipped, lower-fat mixture). Finally, if you're trying to reduce the fat overall, applesauce can be substituted for part of these cookies' fat. However, I wouldn't replace it entirely, as the results can be overly sweet and a bit dry.

Nutrition:

Calories: 78

Total fat: 4g

Cholesterol: 0mg

Carbohydrates: 11g

Fibre: 1g

Protein: 1g

Easy Cinnamon Crisps

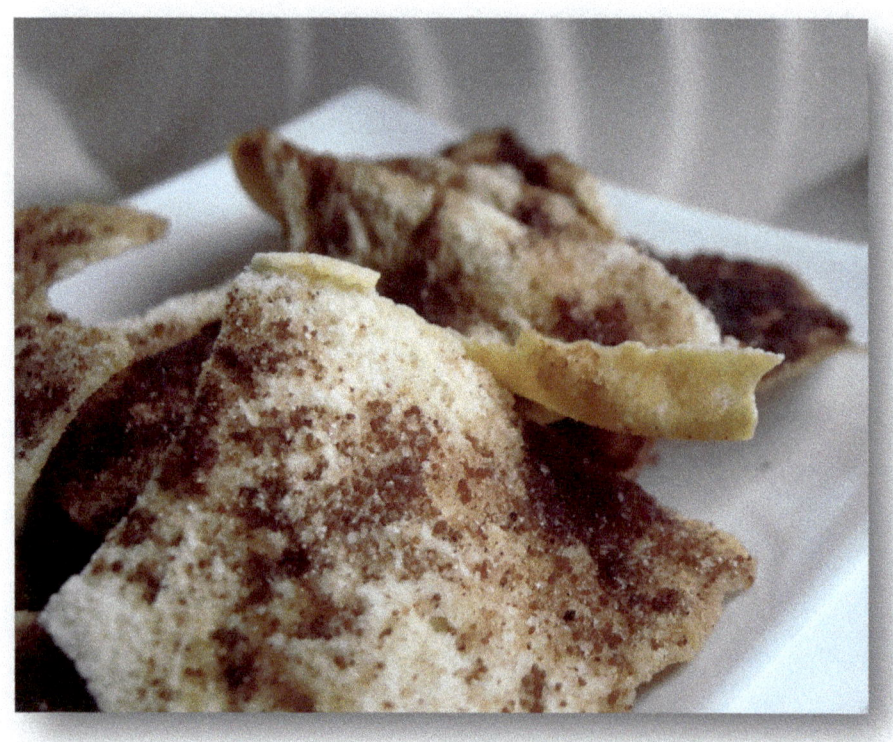

Preparation time: 2 minutes
Cooking time: 6 minutes
Servings: 4
Fry: 347°F

Ingredients:
- 1 (8-inch) tortilla, preferably sprouted whole-grain
- Cooking oil spray it can be (sunflower, safflower, or refined coconut)
- 2 tsp. coconut sugar
- ½ tsp. cinnamon

Directions:

Cut the tortilla into eight triangles (like a pizza). Place on a large plate and spray both sides with oil.

Sprinkle the tops evenly with the coconut sugar and cinnamon. In short, spurts, respray the tops with the oil. (If you spray too hard for this step, it will make the powdery toppings fly off!)

Place directly in the air fryer basket in a single layer (its okay if they overlap a little, but do your best to give them space). Fry and cook for about 5 to 6 minutes, or until the triangles are lightly browned, but not too brown—they're bitter if overcooked. Enjoy warm if possible.

Nutrition:

Calories: 45

Total fat: 1g

Cholesterol: 0mg

Carbohydrates: 8g

Fibre: 1g

Protein: 1g

De-Light-Full Caramelized Apples

Preparation time: 4 minutes
Cooking time: 20 minutes
Servings: 2
Bake: 392°F

Ingredients:

- Two apples, any sweet variety
- 2 tbsp. water
- 1½ tsp. coconut sugar
- ¼ tsp. cinnamon
- Pinch nutmeg
- Dash sea salt
- Cooking oil spray it can be (sunflower, safflower, or refined coconut)

Directions:

Cut each apple in half (no need to peel) and then remove the core and seeds, doing your best to keep the apple halves intact—because ideally, you want apple halves, not quarters.

Place the apples upright in a 6-inch round, 2-inch deep baking pan. Add about two tbsp. of water at the bottom of the dish to keep the apples from drying out (the apples will sit in the water).

With sugar, cinnamon, and nutmeg, dust the tops of the apples evenly. Give each half a very light sprinkle of sea salt.

Spray the tops with oil (if you spray too hard, it will make the toppings fly off in a tragic whirlwind). Once moistened, sprinkle the tops again with oil. (This will keep them from drying out.)

Bake and cook for 20 minutes, or until the apples are very soft and nicely browned on top. Enjoy immediately, plain or topped with granola and ice cream.

Nutrition:

Calories: 120

Total fat: 1g

Cholesterol: 0mg

Carbohydrates: 33g

Fibre: 6g

Protein: 1g

Vegan Snacks

Beets Chips

Preparation time: 10 minutes
Cooking time: 20 minutes
Servings: 4

Ingredients:
- Cooking spray
- Four medium beets, peeled and cut into skinny slices
- Salt and black pepper to the taste
- 1 tbsp. chives, chopped

Directions:
Arrange beets chips in your air fryer's basket, grease with cooking spray, season with salt and black pepper, cook them at 350 degrees F for 20 minutes, flipping them halfway, transfer to bowls and serve with chives sprinkled on top as a snack
Enjoy!

Nutrition:
Calories 80
Fat 1g
Fiber 2g
Carbs 6g
Protein 1g

Avocado Chips

Preparation time: 10 minutes
Cooking time: 10 minutes
Servings: 3

Ingredients:
- One avocado, pitted, peeled and sliced
- Salt and black pepper to the taste
- ½ cup vegan breadcrumbs
- A drizzle of olive oil

Directions:
In a bowl, mix breadcrumbs with salt and pepper and stir.
Brush avocado slices with the oil, coat them in breadcrumbs, place them in your air fryer's basket and cook at the temperature of 390 degrees F for 10 minutes, shaking halfway.
Divide into bowls and serve them as a snack
Enjoy!

Nutrition:
Calories 180
Fat 11g
Fiber 3g
Carbs 7g
Protein 4g

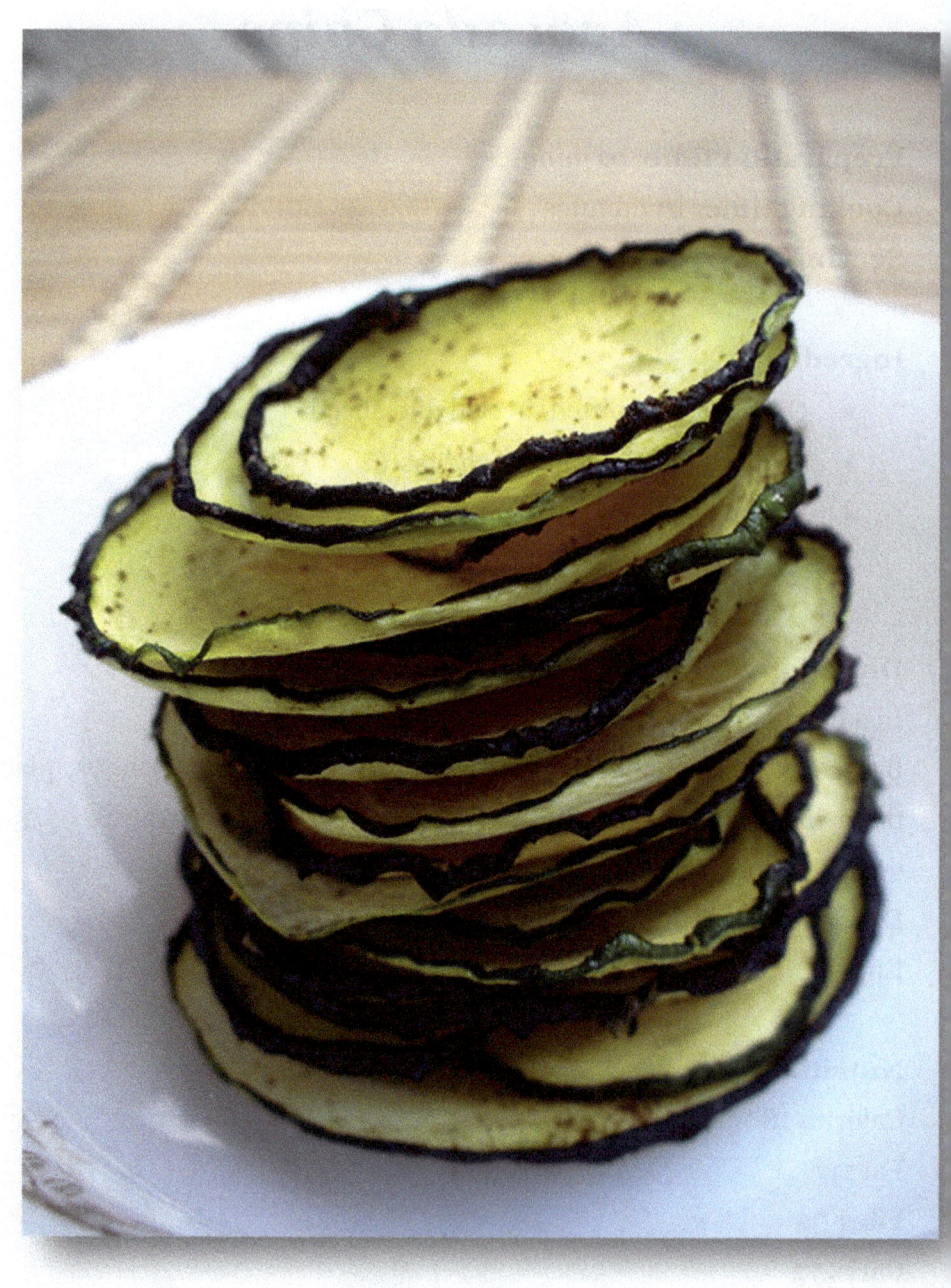

Veggie Sticks

Preparation time: 10 minutes
Cooking time: 30 minutes
Servings: 4

Ingredients:
- Four parsnips, cut into thin sticks
- Two sweet potatoes, cut into sticks
- Four carrots, cut into sticks
- Salt and black pepper to the taste
- 2 tbsp. rosemary, chopped
- 2 tbsp. olive oil
- A pinch of garlic powder

Directions:

Put parsnips, sweet potatoes and carrots in a bowl, add oil, garlic powder, salt, pepper, rosemary, and toss to coat.

Put sweet potatoes in your preheated air fryer, cook them for 10 minutes at 350 degrees F and transfer them to a platter.

Add parsnips to your air fryer, cook for 5 minutes and transfer over potato fries.

Add carrots, cook for 15 minutes at 350 degrees F, also transfer to the platter.

Serve as a snack.

Enjoy!

Nutrition:

Calories 140

Fat 0g

Fiber 2g

Carbs 7g

Protein 4g

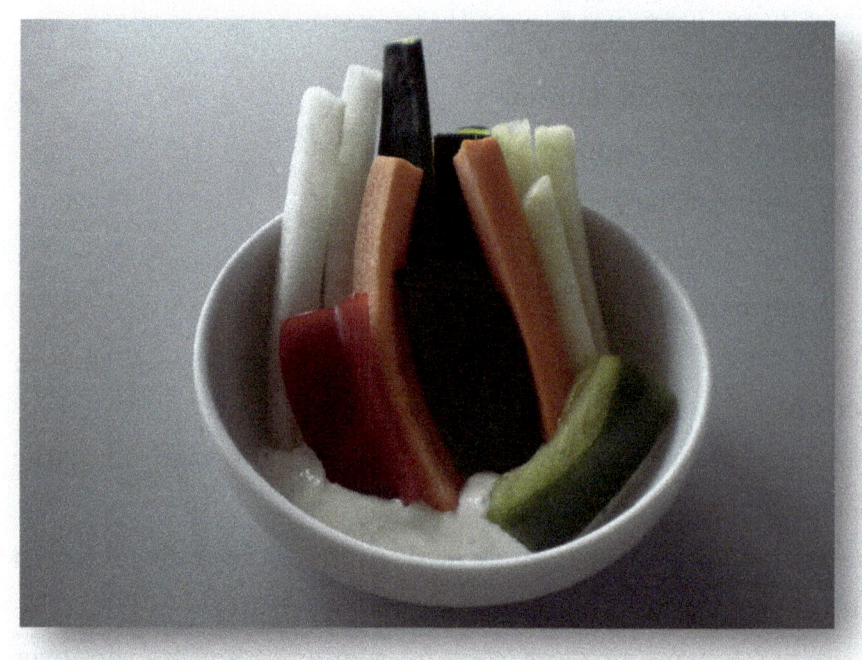

Polenta Biscuits

Preparation time: 10 minutes
Cooking time: 25 minutes
Servings: 4

Ingredients:
- 18 ounces cooked polenta roll, cold
- 1 tbsp. olive oil

Directions:
Cut polenta into medium slices and brush them with the olive oil.
Place polenta biscuits into your air fryer and cook at 400 degrees F for 25 minutes, flipping them after 10 minutes.
Serve biscuits as a snack.

Nutrition:
Calories 120
Fat 0g
Fiber 3g
Carbs 7g
Protein 3g

Vegan Bread and Pizza

Banana Chocolate Muffins

Preparation time: 5 minutes
Cooking time: 20 minutes
Servings: 1-2

Ingredients:

- 1/3 cup oil
- 1/3 lb. brown sugar
- Three ripe bananas
- ½ lb. flour
- 3 tsp. yeast
- ½ lb. chocolate and hazelnut cream

Directions:

Peel the bananas and chop them. Put them in a bowl and cook them with the help of a fork. Add the oil, sugar and stir until everything is integrated.

Add the flour with the yeast sifted and continue stirring until you obtain a homogeneous dough.

Arrange muffin capsules on the plate and fill them with the batter to 2/3 full. Pour 1 tsp of cocoa cream on top and stir with a toothpick to blend well.

Bake and cook the muffins for 20 minutes in the air fryer preheated to 360 degrees F until they are done. Remove and cool on a wire rack. Add more chocolate, if you like.

Nutrition:
Calories: 133.1
Carbohydrates: 26.3g
Fat: 2.9g
Protein: 2.4g
Sugar: 6.3g
Cholesterol: 13mg

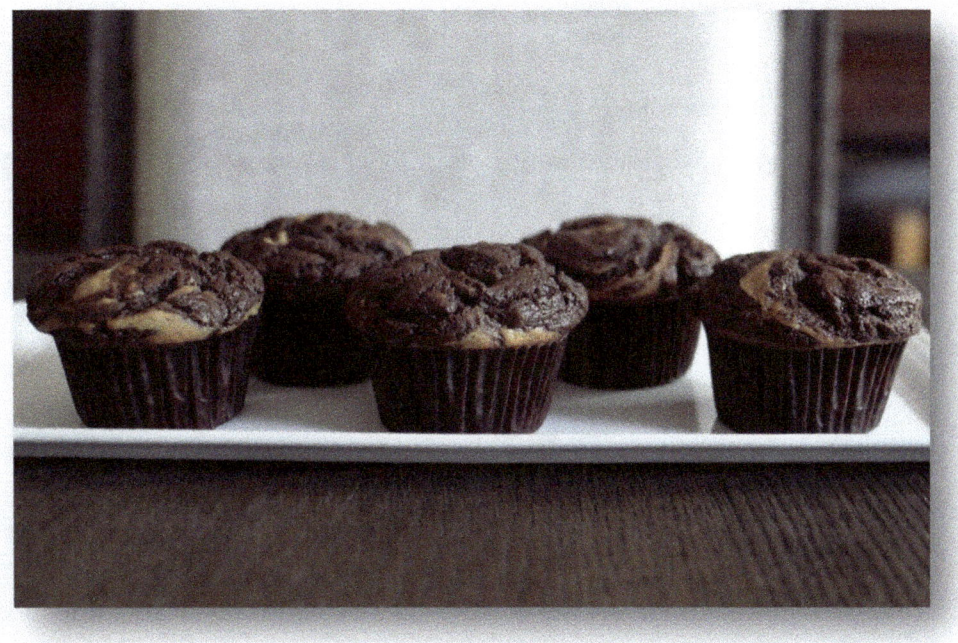

Vegan Corn Bread

Preparation time: 10 minutes
Cooking time: 25 minutes
Servings: 9

Ingredients:
- 1 cup white flour
- 1 cup polenta
- ½ cup brown sugar
- ¼ tsp of salt
- ½ tsp baking soda
- 1 tbsp. baking powder
- ¼ cup of melted butter
- 2 flax eggs
- Vegan buttermilk
- 1/3 cup unsweetened non-dairy milk

Directions:
Preheat the air fryer to 400°F.
In a large bowl, add the white flour, cornmeal, sugar, salt, bicarbonate, yeast, and stir until they are integrated.
Put the rest of the Ingredients to the bowl. Stir again until all the Ingredients have been perfectly integrated.
Pour the dough into a pre-greased baking dish and bake for about 25 minutes or until done. Brown on the outside, and when you put a knife, it comes out clean.

Take the cornbread out of the oven and let it cool for a few minutes before slicing and serving. It can be good to eat hot or cold with vegan butter, maple syrup, jam, substitute for bread, or whatever you like. The leftovers can also be kept in an airtight jar at room temperature or the fridge for about one week or in the freezer for 2 to 3 months.

Nutrition:
Calories: 68.7
Carbohydrates: 13.1g
Fat: 0.7g
Protein: 1.7g
Sugar: 2g
Cholesterol: 0mg

Vegan Banana Bread

Preparation time: 15 minutes
Cooking time: 65 minutes
Servings: 12

Ingredients:
- Three very ripe bananas
- 2 cups of whole wheat flour
- ¾ cup brown sugar
- 1 tsp. ground cinnamon
- 1 tsp. baking soda
- ¼ tsp. of salt
- One flax egg
- ½ cup unsweetened non-dairy milk
- 1/3 cup coconut oil, melted
- 1 tsp. vanilla extract, optional

Directions:

Preheat the air fryer to 350°F.

Using a fork, you can mash the bananas. I recommend that you use cups or a scale to measure the amount of banana because the size of one to another can vary. Use 1 ½ cups. Reserve.

In a bowl, mix flour, sugar, cinnamon, baking soda and salt until they are well integrated.

Add the bananas, flax egg, milk, oil and vanilla extract. Stir until well-integrated.

Grease a pan or line with parchment paper and bake for about 60-70 minutes or until golden brown.

Take out the banana bread and leave it in the mould for at least 15 minutes, then you can move it to a wire rack. Ideally, let it cool completely before slicing it, but you can also have it hot if you want.

Nutrition:

Calories: 209.3

Carbohydrates: 43.4g

Fat: 3.1g

Protein: 2.9g

Sugar: 20.4g

Cholesterol: 0mg

Vegan Bread with Lentils and Unleavened Millet

Preparation time: 25 minutes
Cooking time: 45 minutes
Servings: 2-4

Ingredients:
- 1 lb. coral lentils
- ½ lb. of millet
- 1 tbsp. of vinegar or lemon
- 1 tsp. salt
- Water
- Spices to taste (turmeric, ginger, pepper, etc.)

Directions:
Place the lentils and millet in a bowl. Cover them with water and then let stand for 12 hours. After that time, rinse the grains, discarding the soaking water.

Crush the lentils and millet with a mini primer or food processor to form a sticky dough. Add the vinegar or the lemon, the salt and the chosen spices and mix.

Let the dough rest in a bowl and then covered with plastic wrap or with a kitchen cloth at room temperature for two days. After that time, the dough begins to rise, and you will feel an acidic smell due to the grains' fermentation. Place the dough in a previously oiled bread pan or upholstered with vegetable paper.

Take in a preheated air fryer at 360° for about 30-40 minutes or until a toothpick is inserted and it comes out dry.

Nutrition:

Calories: 80

Carbs: 14g

Fat: 2g

Protein: 1g

Vegan Main Dishes

The Easy Paneer Pizza

"Gone Vegan but missing pizza? This is the guilty-free pizza that you need for your vegan journey!"

Preparation time: 5 minutes
Cooking time: 9 minutes
Servings: 4
Temperature: 347degreesF

Ingredients:
- Cooking oil spray as needed
- One flour tortilla sprouted
- ¼ cup vegan pizza sauce
- ½ cup vegan cheese
- Vegan-friendly topping of your choice

Directions:
Preheat your Air Fryer 347 Degrees F
Spray your Air Fryer cooking basket with oil, add tortilla to your Air Fryer basket and pour the sauce in the center
Evenly distribute your topping on top alongside vegan chees e
Bake for 9 minutes
Serve and enjoy!

Nutrition:

Calories: 210

Fat: 6g

Carbohoydrates: 33g

Protein: 5g

Cauliflower Sauce and Pasta

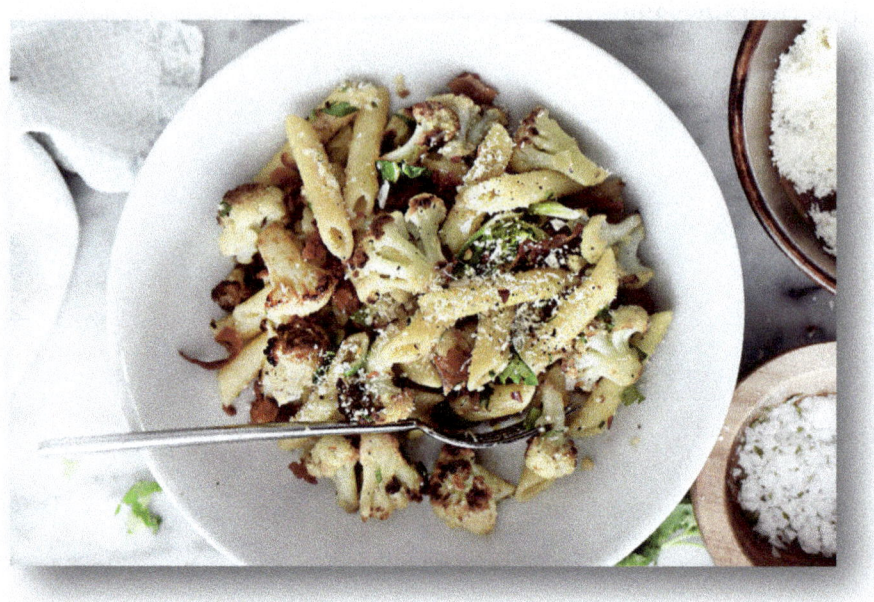

"The vegan pasta for those who are missing the classic Alfredo pasta!"

Preparation time: 10 minutes
Cooking time: 18 minutes
Servings: 4
Temperature: 392degreesF

Ingredients:
- 4 cups cauliflower florets
- Cooking oil as needed
- One medium onion, chopped

- 8 ounces pasta of your choice
- Fresh chives for garnish
- ½ cup cashew pieces
- One and ½ cups of water
- 1 tbsp. Nutritional yeast
- Two large garlic cloves, peeled
- 2 tbsp. fresh lemon juice
- One and ½ tsp. salt
- ¼ tsp. fresh ground black pepper

Directions:
Preheat your Air Fryer 392 Degrees F
Add cauliflower to your Air Fryer basket and spray oil on top. Add onion
Roast for 8 minutes and stir, roast for 10 minutes more
Cook the pasta according to package instructions
Take a blender and add roasted cauliflower and onions alongside cashews, water, yeast, garlic, lemon, garlic, salt, pepper and blend well
Serve pasta together with the sauce on top and a garnish of minced chives and scallions
Serve and enjoy!

Nutrition:
Calories: 341
Fat: 9g
Carbohoydrates: 51g
Protein: 14g

Tamarind Glazed Sweet Potatoes

"If you like the tanginess of tamarind, these tamarind glazed potatoes are what you need!"

Preparation time: 5 minutes
Cooking time: 22 minutes
Servings: 4
Temperature: 395degreesF

Ingredients:
- Five garnet sweet potatoes, peeled and diced
- 1/3 tsp. white pepper
- A few drops of liquid stevia
- 1 tbsp. vegan butter, melted
- 2 tsp. tamarind paste
- ½ tsp. turmeric powder
- One and ½ tbsp. lime juice
- A pinch of the ground allspice

Directions:
Preheat and set the Air Fryer's temperature to 395 degrees F. Get a mixing bowl and add all Ingredients into it.

Mix them until sweet potatoes are well coated. Cook for 12 minutes

Pause the Air Fryer and toss again. Increase the temperature to 390 degrees F

Cook for 10 minutes more

Serve warm and enjoy!

Nutrition:

Calories: 103

Fat: 9.1g

Carbohoydrates: 4.9g

Protein: 1.9g

Vegan Staples

Thai-Inspired Barbecue Cauliflower

Preparation time: 15 minutes
Cooking time: 22 minutes
Servings: 4

Ingredients:

- One large or two small head cauliflower
- One lemon, zest only
- One lime, zest only
- 1 tbsp. brown sugar
- 1/2 cup pumpkin seeds
- Ten garlic cloves
- 1-2 tbsp. Sriracha
- 2 tbsp. curry powder
- 3 tbsp. arrowroot starch or cornstarch
- 3/4 cup coconut milk
- Hot rice, for serving
- Raw vegetables, for serving, optional
- Sea salt, to taste

Directions:

Put the curry, cornstarch, garlic, coconut milk, zest, sugar, sriracha, and salt to taste into a small-sized blender, and then blend until the mixture smooth.

Slice the cauliflower into florets and then put it into a large-sized bowl. Add the curry mixture, toss to coat well, and let marinate for 10 minutes.

Put 1/2 of the marinated cauliflower into the air fryer basket. Set the temperature to 360F and set the timer for 15 minutes, basting every 5 minutes.

Adjust the temperature to 390F, set the timer for 5 to 8 minutes, and cook until crisp. When there are only 2 minutes of cooking, add 1/2 of the air fryer's pumpkin seeds.

Repeat the process with the remaining marinated cauliflower and pumpkin seeds.

Serve with raw veggies, such as celery sticks and carrots, or with hot rice.

Nutrition:

Energy (calories): 190 kcal

Protein: 8.17 g

Fat: 9.51 g

Carbohydrates: 21.8 g

Stuffed Garlic Mushrooms

Preparation time: 10 minutes
Cooking time: 25 minutes
Servings: 4

Ingredients:
- 16 small-sized button mushrooms
- For the stuffing:
- 1 1/2 slices white bread
- 1 1/2 tbsp. olive oil
- One garlic clove, crushed
- 1 tbsp. parsley, flat-leafed, finely chopped
- Ground black pepper, to taste

Directions:
Preheat the air fryer to 390F.
In a food processor, put the bread and process it into fine crumbs. Add the parsley, garlic, and season with pepper to taste. Mix until combined. When thoroughly incorporated, add stir in the olive oil.
Cut the mushroom stalks off and then fill the caps with the breadcrumb mixture, patting the breadcrumb mixture into the lids to make sure no loose crumbs get into the air fryer fan. Put the filled mushroom caps in the air fryer basket, slide the basket back into the housing, cook for about 7-8 minutes or until the mushroom caps are crispy and golden.

Nutrition:

Energy (calories): 82 kcal

Protein: 2.49 g

Fat: 5.47 g

Carbohydrates: 6.59 g

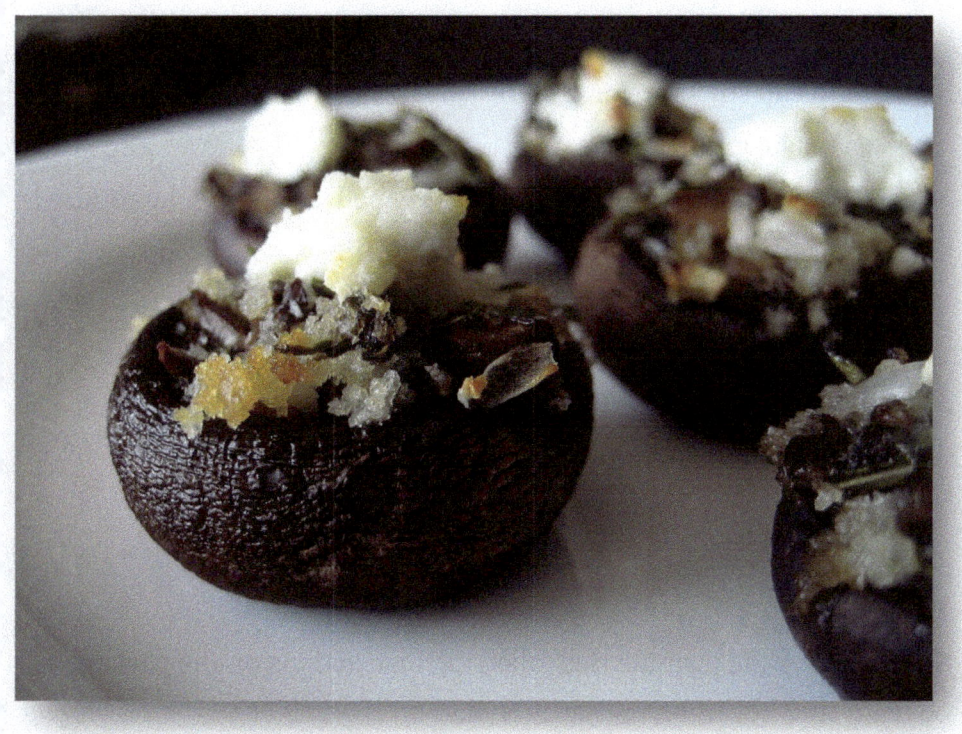

Sticky Mushroom Rice

Preparation time: 5 minutes
Cooking time: 20 minutes
Servings: 6

Ingredients:
- 1/2 cup frozen peas
- 1/2 cup soy sauce or tamari
- 1/2 tsp. ground ginger
- 16 ounces cremini mushrooms, wiped clean, OR large sized mushrooms cut into halves
- 16 ounces jasmine rice, uncooked
- 2 tsp. Chinese five-spice
- Four cloves garlic, finely chopped
- 4 tbsp. maple syrup
- 4 tbsp. white wine or rice vinegar

Directions:
Start cooking the jasmine rice following instructions on the package to be ready and hot when the sauce cooks.

Mix the soy sauce, maple syrup, garlic, five-spice, ground ginger, and white wine until combined. Set aside.

Put the mushrooms in the air fryer basket. Turn the temperature to 350 degrees F and also set the timer for 10 minutes.

Open the air fryer and shake the basket. Pour the soy sauce mixture over the mushroom and add the peas. Stir and cook for 5 minutes.

Pour the mushroom mixture over the pot of rice and stir to mix. Serve.

Nutrition:

Energy (calories): 367 kcal

Protein: 9.49 g

Fat: 5.4 g

Carbohydrates: 79.96 g

Crispy Tofu

Preparation time: 35 minutes
Cooking time: 18 minutes
Servings: 2

Ingredients:
- 2 tbsp. soy sauce, OR tamari for gluten-fre e
- 2 tbsp. Nutritional yeast
- 1/2 tsp. garlic powder
- 1 tsp. water
- 1 tsp. sesame oil
- 1 tbsp. brown rice flour
- One package (8-ounce) firm tofu, rinsed, drained, and then cubed

Directions:

In a small-sized bowl, combine all of the dry Ingredients. Add the wet Ingredients and stir to combine.

Pour the mixture over the tofu cubes, toss to coat, and let marinate for 30 minutes.

After marinating, sprinkles drain excess marinade. Sprinkle the tofu with 1 tbsp. Rice flour and mix to coat. Transfer to the air fryer basket. Turn the temperature to 350 degrees F and set the timer for 18 minutes.

Nutrition:

Energy (calories): 102 kcal

Protein: 5.57 g

Fat: 5.3 g

Carbohydrates: 8.22 g

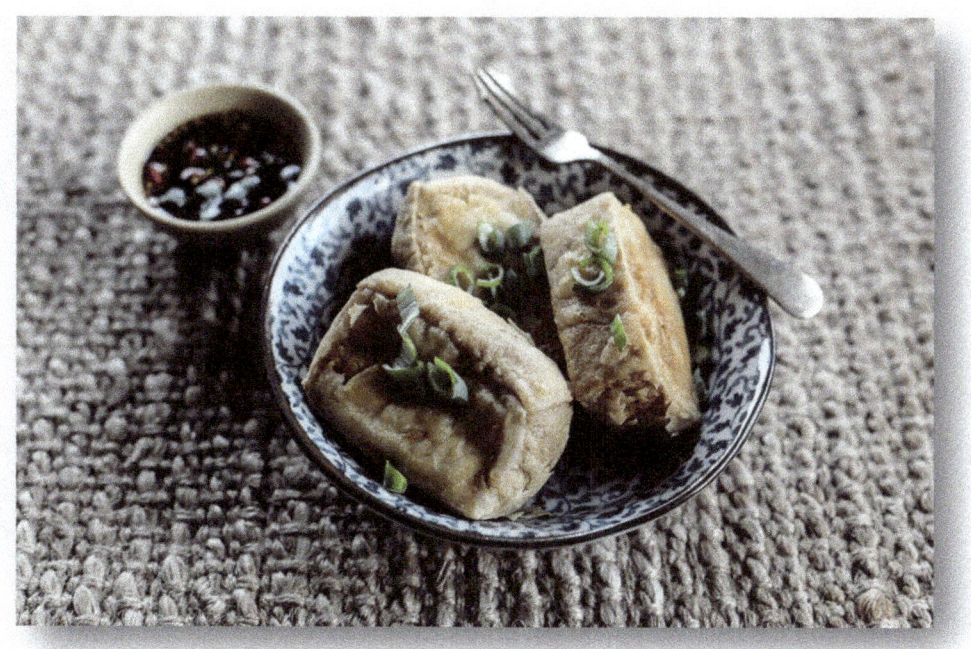

www.ingramcontent.com/pod-product-compliance
Lightning Source LLC
Chambersburg PA
CBHW070733030426
42336CB00013B/1958